PUBLIC HEALTH IN THE 21ST CENTURY SERIES

MEDICARE ADVANTAGE: THE ALTERNATE MEDICARE PROGRAM

PUBLIC HEALTH IN THE 21ST CENTURY SERIES

Family History of Osteoporosis
Afrooz Afghani (Editor)
2009. ISBN: 978-1-60876-190-6

Cross Infections: Types, Causes and Prevention
Jin Dong and Xun Liang (Editors)
2009. ISBN: 978-1-60741-467-4

Health-Related Quality of Life
Erik C. Hoffmann (Editor)
2009. ISBN: 978-1-60741-723-1

Swine Flu and Pig Borne Diseases
Viroj Wiwanitkit
2009. ISBN: 978-1-60876-291-0

Home Fire Safety: Preventive Measures and Issues
Cornelio Moretti (Editor)
2009. ISBN: 978-1-60741-651-7

Biological Clocks: Effects on Behavior, Health and Outlook
Oktav Salvenmoser and Brigitta Meklau (Editors)
2010. ISBN: 978-1-60741-251-9

Sexual Risk Behaviors
Luigi Passero and Cecilia Sgariglia (Editors)
2010. ISBN: 978-1-60741-227-4

MRSA (Methicillin Resistant Staphylococcus aureus) Infections and Treatment
Manal M. Baddour
2010. ISBN: 978-1-61668-038-1

MRSA (Methicillin Resistant Staphylococcus aureus) Infections and Treatment
Manal M. Baddour
2010. ISBN: 978-1-61668-450-1 (Online Book)

Infectious Disease Modelling Research Progress
Jean Michel Tchuenche and C. Chiyaka (Editors)
2010. ISBN: 978-1-60741-347-9

Expedited Partner Therapy in the Management of STDs
H. Hunter Handsfield, Matthew Hogben, Julia A. Schillinger, Matthew R. Golden, Patricia Kissinger, and P. Frederick Sparling
2010. ISBN: 978-1-60741-571-8

Firefighter Fitness: A Health and Wellness Guide
Ernest L. Schneider
2010. ISBN: 978-1-60741-650-0

The Making of a Good Doctor
B. D. Kirkcaldy, R. J. Shephard and R. G. Siefen
2010. ISBN: 978-1-60876-449-5

Handbook of Disease Outbreaks: Prevention, Detection and Control
Albin Holmgren and Gerhard Borg (Editors)
2010. ISBN: 978-1-60876-224-8

Avian Influenza: Etiology, Pathogenesis and Interventions
Salomon Haugan and Walter Bjornson (Editors)
2010. ISBN: 978-1-60741-846-7

Overweightness and Walking
Caleb I. Black (Editor)
2010. ISBN: 978-1-60741-298-4

Overweightness and Walking
Caleb I. Black (Editor)
2010. ISBN: 978-1-61668-516-4
(Online Book)

Smoking Relapse: Causes, Prevention and Recovery
Johan Egger and Mikel Kalb (Editors)
2010. ISBN: 978-1-60876-580-5

Diabetes in Women
Eliza I. Swahn (Editor)
2010. ISBN: 978-1-61668-692-5

Diabetes in Women
Eliza I. Swahn (Editor)
2010. ISBN: 978-1-61668-801-1
(Online Book)

Sepsis: Symptoms, Diagnosis and Treatment
Joseph R. Brown (Editor)
2010. ISBN: 978-1-60876-609-3

Sepsis: Symptoms, Diagnosis and Treatment
Joseph R. Brown (Editor)
2010. ISBN: 978-1-61668-448-8
(Online Book)

Strategic Implications for Global Health
Maria Labonté (Editor)
2010. ISBN: 978-1-60741-660-9

Health and Environment: Social Science Perspectives
Helen Kopnina and Hans Keune (Editors)
2010. ISBN: 978-1-60876-216-3

The Anti-Inflammatory Effects of Exercise
Pedro Tauler and Antoni Aguiló
2010. ISBN: 978-1-60876-886-8

Treating Tobacco Dependence in Vulnerable Populations
John E. Snyder and Megan J. Engelen
2010. ISBN: 978-1-60876-976-6

Controlling Disease Outbreaks: The Changing Role of Hospitals
Raoul E. Nap, Nico E.L. Meessen, Maarten P.H.M. Andriessen, and Tjip S. van der Werf
2010. ISBN: 978-1-61668-314-6

Controlling Disease Outbreaks: The Changing Role of Hospitals
Raoul E. Nap, Nico E.L. Meessen, Maarten P.H.M. Andriessen, and Tjip S. van der Werf
2010. ISBN: 978-1-61668-739-7
(Online Book)

The H1N1 Influenza Pandemic of 2009
Charles R. Bartolotti (Editor)
2010. ISBN: 978-1-61668-357-3

The H1N1 Influenza Pandemic of 2009
Charles R. Bartolotti (Editor)
2010. ISBN: 978-1-61668-392-4
(Online Book)

Heavy Metals: A Rapid Clinical Guide to Neurotoxicity and other Common Concerns
Kenneth R. Spaeth, Antonios J. Tsismenakis and Stefanos N. Kales
2010. ISBN: 978-1-60876-634-5

Physical Activity in Rehabilitation and Recovery
Holly Blake (Editor)
2010. ISBN: 978-1-60876-400-6

Treadmill Exercise and its Effects on Cardiovascular Fitness, Depression and Muscle Aerobic Function
Nuno Azóia and Pedra Dobreiro (Editors)
2010. ISBN: 978-1-60876-857-8

COPD Is/Is Not a Systemic Disease?
Claudio F. Donner (Editor)
2010. ISBN: 978-1-60876-051-0

Research Methodologies in Public Health
David A. Yeboah
2010. ISBN: 978-1-60876-810-3

Diarrhea: Causes, Types and Treatments
Hannah M. Wilson (Editor)
2010. ISBN: 978-1-61668-449-5

Diarrhea: Causes, Types and Treatments
Hannah M. Wilson (Editor)
2010. ISBN: 978-1-61668-874-5
(Online Book)

Medicare Advantage: The Alternate Medicare Program
Charles V. Baylis (Editor)
2010. ISBN: 978-1-60876-031-2

PUBLIC HEALTH IN THE 21ST CENTURY SERIES

MEDICARE ADVANTAGE: THE ALTERNATE MEDICARE PROGRAM

CHARLES V. BAYLIS
EDITOR

Nova Science Publishers, Inc.
New York

For permission to use material from this book please contact us:
Telephone 631-231-7269; Fax 631-231-8175
Web Site: http://www.novapublishers.com

LIBRARY OF CONGRESS CATALOGING-IN-PUBLICATION DATA

Medicare Advantage : the alternate Medicare program / editor, Charles V. Baylis.
p. ; cm.
Includes index.
ISBN 978-1-60876-031-2 (hardcover)
1. Medicare. I. Baylis, Charles V.
[DNLM: 1. Medicare--economics. 2. Fee-for-Service Plans--economics--United States. WT 31 M4853 2009]
RA412.3.M42727 2009
368.4'2600973--dc22

2009035603

Published by Nova Science Publishers, Inc. ✆ New York

CONTENTS

PREFACE

Medicare Advantage (MA) is an alternative way for Medicare beneficiaries to receive covered benefits. Under MA, private health plans are paid a per-person amount to provide all Medicare-covered benefits (except hospice) to beneficiaries who enroll in their plan. As of January 2009, all Medicare beneficiaries had access to an MA plan and 23% of beneficiaries enrolled in one. In general, Medicare Advantage plans offer additional benefits or require smaller co-payments or deductibles than original Medicare. Sometimes beneficiaries pay for these additional benefits through a higher monthly premium, but sometimes they are financed through plan savings. This book highlights the many advantages of the alternative Medicare program. This book consists of public documents which have been located, gathered, combined, reformatted, and enhanced with a subject index, selectively edited and bound to provide easy access.

Chapter 1 - Medicare Advantage (MA) is an alternative way for Medicare beneficiaries to receive covered benefits. Under MA, private health plans are paid a per-person amount to provide all Medicare-covered benefits (except hospice) to beneficiaries who enroll in their plan. Eligible individuals may enroll in an MA plan, if one is available in their area. As of January 2009, all Medicare beneficiaries had access to an MA plan and 23% of beneficiaries enrolled in one. Private plans may use different techniques to influence the medical care used by enrollees. Some plans, such as health maintenance organizations (HMOs) may require enrollees to receive care from a restricted network of medical providers; enrollees may be required to see a primary care physician who will coordinate their care and refer them to specialists as necessary. Other types of private plans, such as private fee-for-service (PFFS) plans, may look more like original Medicare, with fewer restrictions on the providers an enrollee can see and minimal coordination of care.

In general, Medicare Advantage plans offer additional benefits or require smaller co-payments or deductibles than original Medicare. Sometimes beneficiaries pay for these additional benefits through a higher monthly premium, but sometimes they are financed through plan savings. The extent of extra benefits and reduced cost sharing vary by plan type and geography, creating an inequity that can frustrate some beneficiaries. However, Medicare Advantage plans are seen by some as an attractive alternative to more expensive supplemental insurance policies found in the private market.

Though plans that manage their enrollees' care have the potential to be less expensive than original Medicare, recent analyses by the Medicare Payment Advisory Commission (MEDPAC) find that Medicare is projected to pay private plans an average of 14% more per beneficiary in 2009 than it does for beneficiaries in the original Medicare program. While some support the higher Medicare expenditures for MA enrollees because funds are used to provide reduced cost sharing or additional benefits, others support paying private plans no more than the cost of covered benefits under the original Medicare program, which may result in less generous MA benefit packages, or reduced access to MA plans. With competing health expenditure priorities, Congress is likely to examine the MA program.

Congress may consider additional issues. First, the Comparative Cost Adjustment (CCA) Program is slated to start in 2010. CCA is designed to test direct competition between MA and original Medicare. As such, the Part B premiums of beneficiaries in original Medicare may be increased or decreased depending on the efficiency of original Medicare relative to MA plans in the area. Second, recent studies show that profits in 2005 and 2006 for MA plans were, on average, higher than estimated because of underestimates in medical spending. If plans had more accurately estimated future medical spending, they could have offered more generous benefit packages without reducing their profits, though some variability in the accuracy of estimates may be expected. Third, marketing behaviors of MA plans and their agents or brokers were a concern in the 110th Congress; it is unclear whether they will continue to be an issue in the 111th Congress.

The Congressional Budget Office (CBO) March 2008 projection of Medicare payments under Medicare Advantage is $112.8 billion in 2009 for coverage of 11.0 million enrollees, increasing to $221.2 billion in 2018 for 16.6 billion enrollees. This report is an overview of the Medicare Advantage program, and includes legislative history and analysis of recent trends. It will be updated to reflect significant changes to the program.

Chapter 2 - Medicare Advantage (MA) plans are an alternative to the original Medicare fee-for-service (FFS) program. Private fee-for-service (PFFS) plans—one type of MA plan—give beneficiaries an option that is more like Medicare FFS than other MA plans, with a wider choice of providers and less plan management of services and providers. PFFS enrollment increased from about 35,000 beneficiaries in June 2004 to about 2.3 million in June 2008. This report compares PFFS plans to other MA plans and Medicare FFS in three areas: (1) characteristics of beneficiaries, (2) financial risks for beneficiaries who do not contact their plans before receiving services, and (3) disenrollment rates. To do this work, GAO reviewed materials from a selected sample of nine PFFS plan sponsors, analyzed Medicare data, and interviewed officials from CMS, which administers the Medicare program, and other organizations.

Chapter 3 - In 2006, the federal government spent about $59 billion on Medicare Advantage (MA) plans, an alternative to the original Medicare fee-for-service (FFS) program. Although health plans were originally envisioned in the 1980s as a potential source of Medicare savings, such plans have generally increased program spending. Payments to MA plans have been estimated to be 12 percent greater than what Medicare would have spent in 2006 had MA beneficiaries been enrolled in Medicare FFS. Some policymakers are concerned about the cost of the MA program and its contribution to overall spending on the Medicare program, which already faces serious long-term financial challenges.

MA plans receive a per member per month (PMPM) payment to provide services covered under Medicare FFS. Almost all MA plans receive an additional Medicare payment, known as a rebate. Plans use rebates and sometimes additional beneficiary premiums to fund benefits not covered under Medicare FFS, reduce premiums, or reduce beneficiary cost sharing.

This report examines for 2007 (1) MA plans' projected rebate allocations; (2) additional benefits MA plans commonly covered and their costs; (3) MA plans' projected cost sharing; and (4) MA plans' allocation of projected revenues and expenses. GAO analyzed data on MA plans' projected revenues and covered benefits for the most common types of MA plans, accounting for 71 percent of all beneficiaries in MA plans.

To view the full product, including the scope and methodology, click on GAO-08-359. For more information, contact James Cosgrove at (202) 512-7114 or cosgrovej@gao.gov.

Chapter 4 - The federal government's spending on the Medicare Advantage (MA) program has grown substantially in recent years, from approximately $60 billion in 2006 and $77 billion in 2007 to an estimated $91 billion in 2008. MA organizations provide health care coverage to Medicare beneficiaries through private health plans, thus offering an alternative to the original Medicare fee-for-service (FFS) program. Payments to MA organizations are, in part, based on the projected expenditures organizations submit in their bids for providing Medicare-covered services, as well as actual enrollment and beneficiary health status. Once Medicare payments are determined, they are not modified based on differences between actual and projected expenses. MA organizations are not required to submit claims data to the Centers for Medicare & Medicaid Services (CMS)—the agency that administers Medicare—but they must report actual expenditures for the year 2 years prior to the upcoming contract year. For example, MA organizations reported their actual 2006 expenditures in their bid submission for contract year 2008. When MA organizations submit their bids, the actual expenditures reported in their bid submissions reflect the MA organizations' most recent full calendar year of actual expenditure data.

In June 2008, the contributors reported that for 2005, MA organizations generally spent less on medical expenses and earned more profits than projected. MA organizations' self-reported actual profit margin was approximately 5 percent of total revenue, on average, which was approximately $1.1 billion more in 2005 than MA organizations had projected.

The accuracy of MA organizations' projections is important because, in addition to determining Medicare payments, these projections also affect the extent to which MA beneficiaries receive additional benefits not provided under FFS and the amounts beneficiaries pay in cost sharing and premiums. For example, if MA organizations had more accurately projected their revenues and expenses in 2005, they would have been able to provide beneficiaries with additional benefits or cost-sharing reductions, and still maintain the level of profits projected.

This report responds to your request for updated information on the accuracy of MA organizations' projections. Specifically, this report compares MA organizations' 2006 actual medical expenses, non-medical expenses, and profits to projections for the same year, and compares 2006 results to 2005 results. When the contributors requested data from CMS, 2006 was the most recent year for which data were available.

To report MA organizations' actual expenditures, actual profits and projections for 2006, we analyzed the two-year look-back form that MA organizations submitted in 2007 to CMS with the 2008 Bid Pricing Tool. The 2008 two-year look-back form contains MA organizations' selfreported actual medical expenses, non-medical expenses, and profits for 2006, in addition to the projections for 2006 the organizations submitted in 2005. MA organizations submit a single two-year look-back form for each of their contracts, which may include more than one health benefit plan. The contributors excluded employer group health plans because these plans are not open to the general Medicare population, and actual and projected expenses are calculated differently than for other plans. The contributors also excluded small contracts, defined as those with fewer than 24,000 "member months" (equivalent to 2,000 beneficiaries enrolled for a full year), because CMS officials stated they do not consider data from these contracts to be fully credible. Additionally, the contributors excluded two contracts for which actual or projected expenditures were missing. After all exclusions, our analysis included 224 contracts, representing about 57 percent of the contracts for which a two-year look-back form was submitted and about 84 percent of MA enrollment, equivalent to approximately 5.6 million beneficiaries enrolled in contracted plans for a full year. Within the contributors sample of contracts, the contributors analyzed data for three different plan types: Health Maintenance Organizations (HMO), Private Fee-for-Service (PFFS) plans, and Preferred Provider Organizations (PPO). These plan types account for 82 percent of enrollment and 55 percent of contracts for which a two-year look-back form was submitted. To determine actual and projected expenses and profits for 2005 and 2006, the contributors multiplied both actual and projected per member per month expenses and profits by actual enrollment in member months for that year. To compute average actual and projected expenses and profits as a percentage of revenue, the contributors weighted each MA organization's percentage by its total revenue. This approach differs slightly from the enrollment weighting approach we used in our June 2008 report, although the two approaches yield nearly identical results. The percentages reported in our June 2008 report are included in the background section. Results are reported for the specific contract year and may not be representative of or generalizable to other contract years.

The contributors interviewed officials at CMS about data reliability and reviewed all data for reasonableness and consistency; while we did not independently audit MA organizations' selfreported data, the contributors were able to determine that the data were sufficiently reliable for our purposes. We conducted this performance audit from October 2008 to November 2008, in accordance with generally accepted government auditing standards. Those standards require that we plan and perform the audit to obtain sufficient, appropriate evidence to provide a reasonable basis for our findings and conclusions based on our audit objectives. The contributors believe that the evidence obtained provides a reasonable basis for our findings and conclusions based on our audit objectives.

Chapter 5 - Medicare provides federal health insurance for 43 million people who are aged or disabled or who have end-stage renal disease. Most receive services through the traditional fee-for-service (FFS) part of the program, which pays providers a set fee for each covered service (or bundle of services). Participants can choose their providers and are not required to obtain prior authorization for any covered service.

Medicare beneficiaries have the option of enrolling in Medicare Advantage—the program through which private plans participate in Medicare—rather than receiving their care through the FFS program.[1] They may choose to do so because such plans provide additional benefits beyond those available within traditional Medicare, including coverage for services not covered by FFS Medicare (for instance, dental services) and cash rebates of premiums or reduced cost-sharing. As of June 2007, about 18 percent of beneficiaries are enrolled in Medicare Advantage plans.[2] This brief describes how those private plans function, how they are paid, how their costs compare with the costs of traditional Medicare, and how those costs vary by geographic area.

In summary:

- Enrollment in Medicare Advantage is growing rapidly, particularly in a relatively unmanaged type of plan called private fee for service (PFFS).
- Medicare's payments for beneficiaries enrolled in Medicare Advantage plans are higher, on average, than what the program would spend if those beneficiaries were in the FFS sector—so shifts in enrollment out of the FFS program and into private plans increase net Medicare spending.
- The difference in costs relative to those for the traditional FFS program is particularly large for PFFS plans.
- The additional cost to the government for Medicare Advantage plans subsidizes the beneficiaries who enroll in such plans, which fuels the plans' growth in enrollment and raises costs for Medicare beneficiaries who do not participate in Medicare Advantage.
- Reducing the payment differential between Medicare Advantage and the FFS program could result in substantial savings to the Medicare program. But it would also diminish the supplemental benefits and cash rebates that Medicare Advantage plans can offer to enrollees and lessen enrollment in those plans. Lowering payments to those plans would slightly reduce the standard premiums for Part B of Medicare (Supplementary Medical Insurance) and delay the exhaustion of the trust fund that supports Part A (Hospital Insurance).

In: Medicare Advantage: The Alternate Medicare … ISBN: 978-1-60876-031-2
Editors: Charles V. Baylis, pp.1-48

Chapter 1

MEDICARE ADVANTAGE

Paulette C. Morgan

SUMMARY

Medicare Advantage (MA) is an alternative way for Medicare beneficiaries to receive covered benefits. Under MA, private health plans are paid a per-person amount to provide all Medicare-covered benefits (except hospice) to beneficiaries who enroll in their plan. Eligible individuals may enroll in an MA plan, if one is available in their area. As of January 2009, all Medicare beneficiaries had access to an MA plan and 23% of beneficiaries enrolled in one. Private plans may use different techniques to influence the medical care used by enrollees. Some plans, such as health maintenance organizations (HMOs) may require enrollees to receive care from a restricted network of medical providers; enrollees may be required to see a primary care physician who will coordinate their care and refer them to specialists as necessary. Other types of private plans, such as private fee-for-service (PFFS) plans, may look more like original Medicare, with fewer restrictions on the providers an enrollee can see and minimal coordination of care.

In general, Medicare Advantage plans offer additional benefits or require smaller co-payments or deductibles than original Medicare. Sometimes beneficiaries pay for these additional benefits through a higher monthly premium, but sometimes they are financed through plan savings. The extent of extra benefits and reduced cost sharing vary by plan type and geography, creating an inequity that can frustrate some beneficiaries. However, Medicare Advantage plans are seen by some as an attractive alternative to more expensive supplemental insurance policies found in the private market.

Though plans that manage their enrollees' care have the potential to be less expensive than original Medicare, recent analyses by the Medicare Payment Advisory Commission (MEDPAC) find that Medicare is projected to pay private plans an average of 14% more per beneficiary in 2009 than it does for beneficiaries in the original Medicare program. While some support the higher Medicare expenditures for MA enrollees because funds are used to provide reduced cost sharing or additional benefits, others support paying private plans no more than the cost of covered benefits under the original Medicare program, which may result in less generous MA benefit packages, or reduced access to MA plans. With competing health expenditure priorities, Congress is likely to examine the MA program.

Congress may consider additional issues. First, the Comparative Cost Adjustment (CCA) Program is slated to start in 2010. CCA is designed to test direct competition between MA and original Medicare. As such, the Part B premiums of beneficiaries in original Medicare may be increased or decreased depending on the efficiency of original Medicare relative to MA plans in the area. Second, recent studies show that profits in 2005 and 2006 for MA plans were, on average, higher than estimated because of underestimates in medical spending. If plans had more accurately estimated future medical spending, they could have offered more generous benefit packages without reducing their profits, though some variability in the accuracy of estimates may be expected. Third, marketing behaviors of MA plans and their agents or brokers were a concern in the 110th Congress; it is unclear whether they will continue to be an issue in the 111th Congress.

The Congressional Budget Office (CBO) March 2008 projection of Medicare payments under Medicare Advantage is $112.8 billion in 2009 for coverage of 11.0 million enrollees, increasing to $221.2 billion in 2018 for 16.6 billion enrollees. This report is an overview of the Medicare Advantage program, and includes legislative history and analysis of recent trends. It will be updated to reflect significant changes to the program.

INTRODUCTION

Medicare Advantage (MA) is an alternative way for Medicare beneficiaries to receive covered benefits. Under MA, private health plans are paid a per-person amount to provide all Medicare covered benefits (except hospice) to beneficiaries who enroll in their plan. Eligible individuals may enroll in an MA plan, if one is available in their area. As of January 2009, all Medicare beneficiaries had access to an MA plan and 23% of beneficiaries enrolled in one. Private plans may use different techniques to influence the medical care used by enrollees. Some plans, such as health maintenance organizations (HMOs) may require enrollees to receive care from a restricted network of medical providers; enrollees may be required to see a primary care physician who will coordinate their care and refer them to specialists as necessary. Other types of private plans, such as private fee-for-service (PFFS) plans, may look more like original Medicare, with fewer restrictions on the providers an enrollee can see and minimal coordination of care.

In general, Medicare Advantage plans offer additional benefits or require smaller co-payments or deductibles than original Medicare. Sometimes beneficiaries pay for these additional benefits through a higher monthly premium, but sometimes they are financed through plan savings. The extent of extra benefits and reduced cost sharing vary by plan type and geography, creating an inequity that can frustrate some beneficiaries. However, Medicare Advantage plans are seen by some as an attractive alternative to more expensive supplemental insurance policies found in the private market.

The 111th Congress may examine several aspects of the MA program. First, Medicare is projected to pay MA plans more per beneficiary than it does for beneficiaries in original Medicare—an effect of a payment formula designed to encourage plan participation. Though a portion of the higher expenditure results in extra benefits and reduced cost sharing for some enrollees, some argue that private plans should not be paid more than the cost of original Medicare. Second, starting in 2010, the Comparative Cost Adjustment (CCA) Program will test direct competition between MA and original Medicare in selected areas. As such, the Part B premiums of beneficiaries in original Medicare may be increased or decreased depending on the efficiency of original Medicare relative to MA plans in the area. Third, recent studies show that profits in 2005 and 2006 for MA plans were, on average, higher than estimated because of underestimates in medical spending. If plans had more accurately estimated medical spending, they could have offered more generous benefit packages without reducing their profits, though some variability in the accuracy of estimates may be expected. Finally, marketing behaviors of MA plans and their agents or brokers were a concern in the 110th Congress; it is unclear whether they will continue to be an issue in the 111th. All of these issues are discussed in more detail in the "Issues for Congress" section at the end of this report.

The Congressional Budget Office (CBO) March 2008 projection of Medicare payments under Part C is $112.8 billion in 2009 for coverage of 11.0 million enrollees, increasing to $221.2 billion in 2018 for 16.6 billion enrollees.

BACKGROUND

Medicare has a long-standing history of offering its beneficiaries health insurance coverage through private plans. Beginning in the 1970s, private health plans were allowed to contract with Medicare on a cost-reimbursement basis. Under a cost contract, plans are reimbursed for the actual costs of delivering health care services. In 1982, Congress passed the Tax Equity and Fiscal Responsibility Act (TEFRA, P.L. 97-248), which created the first Medicare risk contracting program. Under a risk contract, participating health plans are paid a fixed monthly payment per enrollee to furnish all Part A and B Medicare-covered services (except hospice) to beneficiaries. This is in contrast to the original fee-for-service (FFS) Medicare, where Medicare pays providers directly for each item or service delivered.

With the passage of TEFRA, payments to private health plans were set at 95% of the cost of providing Medicare benefits in the original FFS program. FFS costs were measured by units called Average Adjusted Per Capita Costs (AAPCCs). By 1997, 15 years after the start of the risk contract program, Medicare private plans covered more than 5 million beneficiaries, or about 14% of beneficiaries. However, despite its lengthy tenure as the basis for private plan payment, the calculation of AAPCCs was criticized for a number of reasons. Principal among these was that payments fluctuated from year to year and varied widely across the country. In an attempt to remedy this problem, Congress, in the Balanced Budget Act of 1997 (BBA, P.L. 105-33), replaced Medicare's risk contract program with the Medicare+Choice (M+C) program. The BBA substantially restructured the system for setting Medicare payment rates to private plans. By establishing a new payment methodology, Congress hoped to reduce Medicare spending, expand access to managed care options, and decrease variation in payment rates across the country. Under the M+C program, the per capita rate for a payment area was set at the highest of three amounts calculated *for each county*:

- a blended rate, which was a blend of an area-specific (local) rate and a national rate;
- a minimum payment (or floor) rate; or
- a rate reflecting a minimum increase from the previous year's rate.

The blended per capita rate was intended to shift payment amounts away from local (generally county) rates, which reflect the wide variations in fee-for-service costs, toward a national average rate. The floor rate was designed to raise payments in certain counties more quickly than would occur through the blend alone; the minimum increase percentage was to protect counties that would otherwise receive only a small increase (if any). This formula was subject to a budget neutrality provision to keep expenditures from exceeding expected expenditures in the absence of the new formula.

Although the intent of the BBA was to increase access to private plans, particularly in markets where availability was limited or non-existent, the program did not work as well as intended. The goal of controlling Medicare spending may have dampened the interest of private plans to develop new markets and add plan options. Their cautious behavior may have been a reaction to a slowdown in the rate of increase in payments. Among plans, there was also a great deal of uncertainty about the future of the M+C program and the stability of payments to sustain the program. Between 1999 and 2003, private plans left the program or reduced their service areas, affecting thousands of enrollees each year. Some enrollees were able to switch to other private Medicare plans, while others had no M+C plans available to them. Despite a small surge in enrollment initially, the percentage of beneficiaries enrolled in M+C dropped from 17% in 1999 to approximately 12% in 2003. To address the decreased plan participation, the 106th Congress inserted provisions in the Balanced Budget Refinement Act of 1999 (BBRA, P.L. 106-113) and the Medicare, Medicaid, and SCHIP Benefits, Improvements, and Protection Act of 2000 (BIPA, P.L. 106-554) to increase reimbursement to M+C plans.

In 2003, Congress passed the Medicare Prescription Drug, Improvement, and Modernization Act of 2003 (MMA, P.L. 108-173), which made substantial changes to Medicare's private plan option. In creating Medicare Advantage (MA) to replace the M+C program, the MMA established an entirely new payment methodology to pay private plans. Under the new payment system, Medicare continues to pay plans a fixed monthly amount per enrollee, but these monthly payments are determined, at least in part, by competitive bidding. In addition, Congress increased payments to plans and introduced regional Preferred Provider Organizations—a popular option in the private health insurance market. Finally, the MMA created a new benefit package for Medicare enrollees: beginning in 2006, beneficiaries have been able to enroll in a Medicare Part D prescription drug plan whether they are in original Medicare or Medicare Advantage. In general, a beneficiary who wants to enroll in an MA plan and receive Part D prescription drug coverage must enroll in an MA-PD plan—an MA plan that includes the Part D coverage. A beneficiary who wants to remain in original Medicare may only enroll in Part D through a Prescription Drug Plan (PDP).

Today Medicare beneficiaries can choose to enroll in several different types of private plans. These include coordinated care plans, also known as managed care plans, such as health maintenance organizations (HMOs), preferred provider organizations (PPOs), and provider sponsored organizations (PSOs) as well as plans that do not manage or coordinate the health care of enrollees, such as private fee-for-service organizations (PFFS) and medical savings accounts (MSA). Certain other plan types operate under exceptions or demonstration authority and may or may not manage care. Not all types are available in all locations.

Prior to the passage of MMA, enrollment in private plans fluctuated. Since the passage of the MMA, overall enrollment in private plans has been steadily increasing. In 2009, approximately 10.4 million, or 23%, of Medicare beneficiaries are enrolled in a MA plan, and all Medicare beneficiaries have access to at least one private plan. Despite these successes, reforming the payment methodology for private plans remains a key issue among policymakers. According to the Medicare Payment Advisory Commission (MEDPAC), Medicare is expected to pay private plans an average of 14% more per beneficiary in 2009 than it does for beneficiaries enrolled in the original Medicare program.[1] A comparable analysis for 2008 showed that Medicare was expected to pay private plans an average of 13% more per beneficiary in 2008 than it did for beneficiaries enrolled in original Medicare.[2] Based on the 2008 analysis, the greater expected payments to plans relative to spending in original Medicare varies by plan type; payments to HMOs are approximately 112% of original Medicare, while payments to PFFS plans are 117% of original Medicare. Since MA payments are based, in part, on historical payment rates, this 13% difference is linked to the 1997 BBA legislation, which created payment floors to attract private plans to certain counties, particularly rural counties. These floors, which exceeded FFS spending levels in many areas, continue to be used in the calculation of MA payment rates today. MA plans use these payments to provide extra benefits to enrollees, but the value of these benefits vary across plan types and across counties. In addition, these higher payments have attracted private plans to areas previously underserved by Medicare private plans, and beneficiaries today have more private plans to choose from than they did 10 years ago.

Current Payment System

Beginning in 2006, the Secretary began determining MA payment rates by comparing plan *bids* to a *benchmark.* By the first week of June each year, plans are required to submit their bids for all MA plans they intend to offer in the upcoming year. Each bid represents the plan's estimated revenue requirement for providing required Parts A and B Medicare services to an average Medicare beneficiary. The revenue requirement includes the estimated cost of providing required health care, plus administrative costs and a return on investment. After plans submit their bids, the Secretary has, with one exception, the authority to negotiate the bid amount, similar to the authority of the Director of the Office of Personnel Management (OPM) with respect to the Federal Employees Health Benefits program. The Secretary's authority to negotiate bids does not extend to bids submitted by Private Fee for Service (PFFS)[3] organizations. The Secretary then compares each plan's bid to a benchmark. The benchmark amounts represent the maximum amount the federal government will pay a plan for providing required Medicare benefits. If a plan's bid is less than the benchmark, its payment equals its bid plus a rebate of 75% of the difference between the benchmark and the bid. The rebate must be used to provide additional benefits to enrollees, reduce Medicare cost sharing expenses, or reduce a beneficiary's monthly Part B, prescription drug, or supplemental premium (for services beyond required Medicare benefits). The remaining 25% of the difference is retained by the federal government. If a plan's bid is equal to or above the benchmark, its payment is equal to the benchmark amount, and each enrollee in that plan will pay an additional premium equal to the amount by which the bid exceeds the benchmark. Any MA plan that provides Part D prescription drug coverage receives reimbursement for premiums and cost-sharing reductions for its qualifying low-income enrollees.

Additional payments may be available to certain types of plans in specific areas, or for enrollment of certain beneficiaries. The MMA increased payments to MA regional plans in three ways. First, the MMA established a regional plan stabilization fund to encourage plans to serve at least one entire region or even all regions, and to encourage plans to stay in regions they might otherwise leave. Originally, $10 billion was to be made available to this fund for years 2007 through 2013, with additional money entering the fund from savings in the regional plan bidding process. However, subsequent legislation reduced the initial $10 billion to one dollar. Money from the regional plan bidding process continues to flow into the fund and will be available for distribution in 2014. Second, the MMA allows the Secretary to provide an increased payment in special circumstances for certain hospitals that provide inpatient hospital services to MA regional plan enrollees. Third, Medicare shared risk with MA regional plans in 2006 and 2007. If a plan's costs fell outside of a specified range or "risk corridor," plans assumed only a portion of the risk for unexpectedly high costs and plans were required to return a portion of the savings to Medicare for unexpectedly low costs.

In general, the MA benchmarks in each local area (county) are updated annually by a minimum increase over the previous year's rate. The minimum increase is set at the larger of either 2% or the overall growth in Medicare expenditures, otherwise known as the National MA Growth Percentage, subject to a budget neutrality adjustment. In certain years (known as *rebasing years*), plan payments are updated by the greater of the minimum increase or 100% of fee-for-service (FFS) costs, with adjustments. Statutorily required adjustments to the 100% of FFS amount include (1) exclusion of the direct cost of medical education, (2) phase-out of the indirect cost of medical education, and (3) adjustment to reflect the additional per capita payments that would have been made in the area if individuals entitled to benefits under Medicare had not received services from the Department of Defense or the Department of Veterans Affairs. (As of CY2009, CMS had been unable to make the third of these adjustments.) According to statute, the Secretary is required to rebase FFS costs at least once every three years. However, CMS has chosen to rebase more frequently. The Secretary opted to rebase FFS rates for 2007 and 2009, but not 2008. In rebasing years, all benchmarks are either equal to or greater than the estimated adjusted average spending in original Medicare in that county. In a non-rebasing year, it is possible for spending in original Medicare in a county to exceed the benchmark amount. But in general, benchmarks are set at or above spending in original Medicare. According to MEDPAC, benchmarks are, on average, 18% greater than expected spending in original Medicare.[4] The National MA Growth Percentage rate (prior to the budget neutrality adjustment discussed below) is 5.7% in 2008 and 4.2% in 2009.

The benchmark is calculated differently for local MA plans than for regional MA plans. The local benchmark is based solely on statutorily or administratively defined increases. The regional benchmark is competitive in that the benchmark consists of two components: a statutorily determined increase and a weighted average of plan bids. The latter component introduces a new form of competition among regional plans, by basing a portion of the benchmark amount on bids submitted by the plans.

After determining the annual update, the Secretary adjusts payments for the health status of enrollees and for budget neutrality. To adjust for health status, the

Secretary calculates a risk score for each enrollee based on the beneficiary's previous health care utilization. (This is known as *risk adjustment.*) Previously, payments to managed care plans were adjusted for a combination of demographic factors such as age, gender, and institutional status. In 1999, Congress urged the Secretary to implement a more clinically based risk adjustment methodology to supplement the existing demographic adjustment factors. It was fully phased in by 2007. The methodology was to be implemented without reducing overall payments to managed care plans. Typically, risk adjustment would have the effect of lowering payments to plans enrolling healthier beneficiaries and raising payments to plans enrolling sicker beneficiaries. To prevent overall payments to managed care plans from going down, the Secretary applied a budget neutrality adjustment. Under budget neutrality, total payments to managed care plans using 100% risk adjusted rates must be equal to total payments to plans using 100% demographic rates. When Congress passed the Deficit Reduction Act of 2005, it included a provision mandating the phaseout of this budget neutrality adjustment by 2011. As a result, the MA benchmark update for 2008 was, on average, 3.5%. The update for 2009 is an average of 3.6% for all areas that did not receive a rebased amount.

MA plans offering prescription drug coverage receive a separate benchmark payment for Part D prescription drug benefits. The benchmark for Part D benefits is based on an adjusted average of all plan bids for the area and is therefore competitively determined.

Trends in Availability and Enrollment

Over time, the number of contracts under MA and its predecessors has fluctuated. From 1987 to the early 1990s, many risk plans terminated existing contracts, decreasing the number of available contracts from 161 in 1987 to 93 in 1991. The number of Medicare risk plans began increasing again in 1992, more than tripling from 110 in 1993 to 346 in 1998. With the implementation of the M+C program in 1999, M+C organizations withdrew from the Medicare program or reduced the size of their service area. As shown in **Figure 1**, the number of contracts dropped from a high of 346 in 1998 to a low of 146 in March 2003. With the passage of the MMA in 2003, the trend began to reverse. The number of MA contracts more than doubled between 2005 and 2006. This increase coincides with the start of the Part D prescription drug program and may reflect an overall increased interest in private plan participation in Medicare at that time. There were 600 MA coordinated care and PFFS contracts in 2008, increasing to 623 in 2009.

Organizations withdrawing from the program or reducing their service area between 1998 and 2004 cited several reasons for leaving the program: inadequate payments, increasing regulatory burden, and difficulty developing or maintaining provider networks. The withdrawals may have reflected strategic business decisions that transcended payment issues. Other factors may have contributed to withdrawals, such as low enrollment and market competition. For each year between January 1999 and January 2003, from 4% to 15% of M+C enrollees either had to change plans or leave the program because of plan withdrawals and service area reductions. Some beneficiaries were required to switch plans multiple times between 1999 and 2003. Of those beneficiaries that lost their plans, between 7% and 24% lost access to any M+C plan each year.

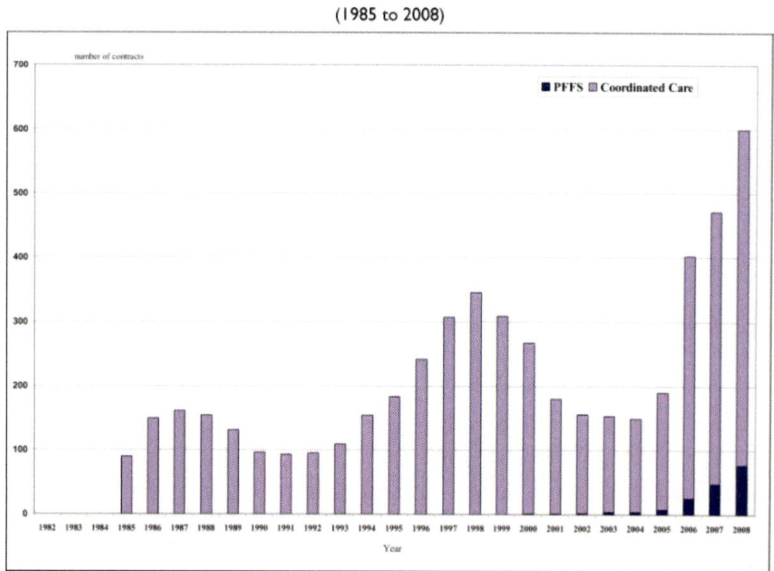

Source: Prepared by the Congressional Research Service based on April CMS Medicare Managed Care Contract (MMCC) Monthly Reports through 2005, and CMS Medicare Advantage Monthly Summary Reports for 2006 to 2008.

Notes: Medicare managed care contracts include risk contracts through 1998, Medicare+Choice contracts beginning in 1999, and Medicare Advantage contracts beginning in 2006. This figure does not contain data for reasonable cost contracts, demonstrations, Health Care Pre Payment (HCPP) plans, PACE plans, Medical Savings Accounts, employer sponsored plans, or pilot projects.

Figure 1. Number of Coordinated Care and PFFS Contracts in Medicare Part C

(selected years, 1985 to 2017)

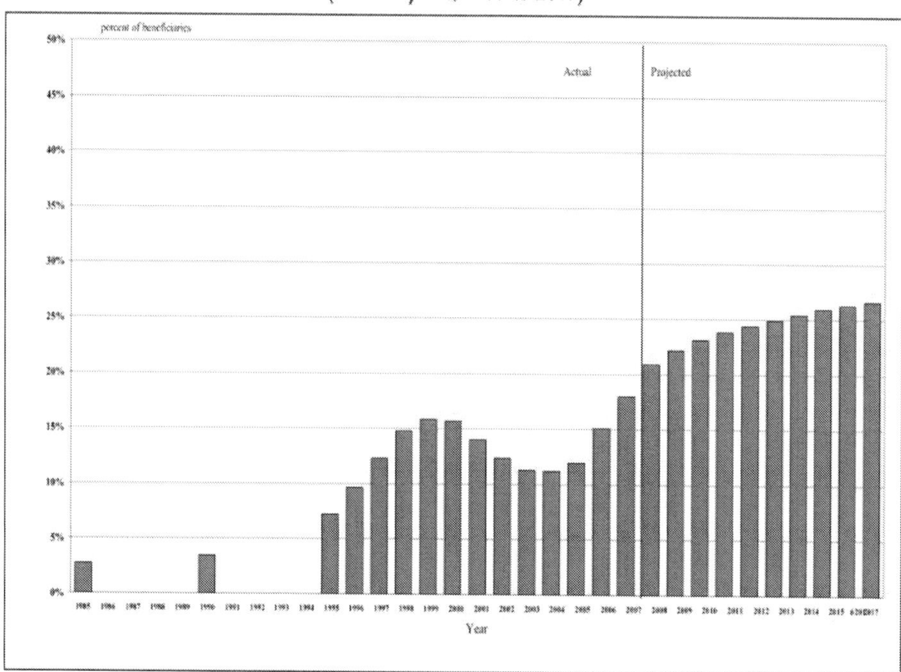

Source: Prepared by CRS based on 2008 Annual Report of the Board of Trustees of the Federal Hospital Insurance and Federal Supplementary Medical Insurance Trust Fund. Enrollment from 2008 to 2015 is estimated.

Notes: Medicare plans include risk plans through 1998, Medicare+Choice plans beginning in 1999, and Medicare Advantage plans beginning in 2006.

Figure 2. Percentage of Beneficiaries Enrolled in Medicare Private Plans, Actual and Projected.

Enrollment in Medicare private plans has fluctuated over time. As shown in **Figure 2**, in 1990 about 3% of Medicare beneficiaries were enrolled in the program, but by 1998 this figure had increased to 15% of Medicare beneficiaries, covering just over 6 million enrollees. With the implementation of the M+C program, enrollment increased through 1999, but declined steadily to a low of 11% (4.7 million enrollees) in 2003 and 2004. Enrollment has since increased each year, reaching a recent high of 23% in 2009. The 2008 Annual Report of the Board of Trustees projects further enrollment increases reaching about 27% of all beneficiaries in 2017, covering about 15 million enrollees.

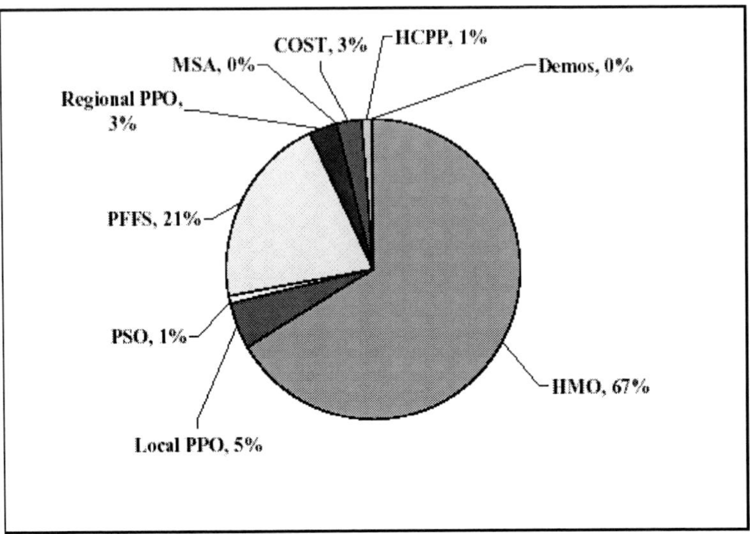

Source: Prepared by CRS based on CMS data.

Notes: HMOs: health maintenance organizations; Local PPO: local preferred provider organizations; PSO: provider sponsored organizations; PFFS: private fee-for-service organizations; Regional PPOs: regional preferred provider organizations; MSA: medical savings accounts; COST: reasonable cost organizations; HCPP: health care pre-payment organizations; Demos: organizations that operate under CMS demonstration authority. May not sum to 100% due to rounding.

Figure 3. Percentage of M.A. Enrollment, by Plan Type, 2008

Plan Type and Enrollment

Though a variety of plan types are authorized under Medicare, national enrollment in MA is concentrated in two types: health maintenance organizations (HMOs), with 67% of enrollment, and private fee-for-service (PFFS) plans, with 21% of enrollment (**Figure 3**). All other remaining plan types make up 13% of enrollment. Characteristics of the different plan types and enrollment specifics follow.

Coordinated Care Plans (CCP)

Coordinated Care Plans (CCPs) are those plans that have a network of medical providers under contract to provide approved health care benefits to plan enrollees. CCPs may use mechanisms to coordinate care or control health care utilization, such as primary care "gatekeepers," and financial incentives with plan providers to encourage cost-effective health care. CCPs include the following specific types of plans: Health Maintenance Organizations (HMOs), Preferred Provider Organizations (PPOs), and Provider Sponsored Organizations (PSOs). Three-quarters of all MA enrollees are in a coordinated care plan.

Health Maintenance Organizations (HMOs)

Health Maintenance Organizations (HMOs) offer services to plan members in designated areas. Beneficiaries are generally required to obtain services from hospitals and doctors in the plan's network. Some plans offer a point-of-service option under which an individual may elect to obtain services from a non-network provider; in such cases, the individual generally pays a greater out of pocket cost for out-of-network care. In 2008, approximately 6 million Medicare beneficiaries (67%) were enrolled in an MA HMO.

Preferred Provider Organizations (PPOs)

A Preferred Provider Organization (PPO) is a plan that has a network of providers; however, enrollees are not restricted to the providers in the PPO network. Generally, enrollees are required to pay greater cost sharing when receiving care outside of the PPO network. Two types of PPO plans are authorized under Medicare: local PPO plans and regional PPO plans. Local PPO plans may choose their service area, while regional PPO plans must agree to serve one or more regions designated by the Secretary. There are 26 PPO regions consisting of states or groups of states. In addition to the service area requirements, the benefit packages for regional PPO plans are required to have a unified Part A and B deductible and a catastrophic out-of-pocket limit, which are not required of local PPO plans. In 2008, 5% of all MA enrollees were in a local PPO plan (approximately 470,000) and 3% of MA enrollees were in a regional PPO plan (approximately 230,000).

Provider Sponsored Organization (PSO)

A Provider Sponsored Organization (PSO) is a coordinated care plan established or organized by a group of medical providers in which the providers furnish the majority of the health care and share in the financial risk of providing the health care to plan enrollees. In 2008, 1% of MA enrollees were in an MA PSO plan (approximately 54,000).

Specialized Plans for Special Needs Individuals (SNPs)

A Specialized Plan for Special Needs Individuals (SNPs) is any MA coordinated care plan that exclusively enrolls or enrolls a disproportionate percentage of special needs individuals. Special needs individuals are any MA eligible individuals who are either institutionalized as defined by the Secretary, eligible for both Medicare and Medicaid, or have a severe or disabling chronic condition and would benefit from enrollment in a specialized MA plan. Since SNP plans may be any type of CCP, SNP enrollees are included in the enrollment estimates above. In 2008, 1.1 million Medicare beneficiaries were enrolled in a SNP: 70% were enrolled in a SNP for beneficiaries eligible for both Medicare and Medicaid, 17% were enrolled in a SNP for beneficiaries with chronic conditions, and 13% were enrolled in a SNP for institutionalized Medicare beneficiaries.

Private Fee for Service plans (PFFS)

Private Fee for Service plans (PFFS) are plans that (1) reimburse hospitals, physicians, and other providers on a fee-for-service basis without placing providers at risk; (2) do not vary rates for a provider based on the utilization relating to that provider; and (3) do not restrict the selection of providers among those who are lawfully authorized to provide services and agree to accept the terms and conditions of payment established by the plan. In 2008, 21% of MA participants were enrolled in a PFFS plan (approximately 1.9 million).

PFFS contracts and enrollment have seen a steeper increase over recent years. First authorized in the BBA, the first contract was offered in 2000, the second following in 2002. However, between 2004 and 2008, MA PFFS contracts grew from 4 contracts in 2004 to 77 contracts in 2008. Enrollment in PFFS grew from 31,550 in 2004 to 1.9 million in 2008. Several factors may have contributed to the recent growth. First, prior to 2011, PFFS contracts are not required to establish provider networks and are therefore less expensive to establish in non-urban areas. Starting in 2011, PFFS plans sponsored by employers or unions will be required to have contracted provider networks. All other PFFS plans will be required to establish provider networks in areas where at least two other network-based plans operate. Second, enrollees can choose to see any provider willing to accept the terms and conditions specified by the PFFS plan—an attractive feature for beneficiaries. Third, PFFS plans tend to be paid more than coordinated care plans. Medicare pays 13% more per beneficiary in MA than in original Medicare. This varies by type of MA plan, with a 12% increase for HMOs and 17% for PFFS. Fourth, PFFS contracts have fewer statutory requirements, resulting in reduced operation costs. And fifth, employer and union groups have historically found MA

PFFS plans an attractive option for providing retiree coverage, though this may change with the new network requirements.

Reasonable Cost Plans (COST)

Reasonable Cost Plans (COST) are private MA plans that are paid on the basis of the reasonable costs actually incurred to provide Medicare covered benefits to enrollees. Unlike other types of private plans that participate in Medicare, Cost plans are not "at risk" for the actual cost of providing care to their enrollees. In 2008, 266,000 beneficiaries were enrolled in a cost plan, representing 3% of total MA enrollment.

Medical Savings Accounts (MSA)

A Medical Savings Account (MSA) under MA is a combination of a health insurance policy with a high deductible and a savings account for health care expenses. CMS pays premiums for the insurance policy and makes contributions to the savings account. Beneficiaries use money from the savings account to pay for their health care before the high deductible of the insurance policy is met. The maximum deductible is set by law. For 2008, the deductible may not exceed $10,050. In 2008, slightly more than 1,000 people were enrolled in an MA MSA. They represented less than 0.01% of MA enrollees.

Health Care Prepayment Plans (HCPP)

A Health Care Prepayment Plan (HCPP) is a private plan that covers only physician services. In 2008, 1% of MA enrollees were in an HCPP in 2008.

Availability by Contract Type

Enrollment in a plan is open only to eligible beneficiaries living in the plan's service area. Plans define a service area as a set of counties and county parts, identified at the zip code level. In 2009, an MA plan is available to every beneficiary in the United States. However, this widespread availability is a recent event. In the early part of the M+C program, a Medicare private plan was not available in the majority of counties (**Table 1**). In 1997, approximately a quarter of counties had an M+C plan available, increasing to 29% by 1999. (In 1997, 76% of counties were without a plan, decreasing to 71% in 1999.) In 2000, the first PFFS plan focused primarily on rural and suburban areas that were less often served by managed care; this greatly increased the proportion of counties with access to a private plan. Between 2001 and 2003, approximately half of counties had access to a PFFS plan, but for over 40% of counties, PFFS was the only private option available. The proportion of counties served by managed care decreased over this period, from 20% of counties in 2001 to 17% of counties in 2003. (In 2001, 10% of all counties were served by only a coordinated care plan, while 10% of all counties were served by both a managed care and a PFFS plan, summing to 20%. In 2003, 9% of all counties were served by only a coordinated care plan, while an additional 8% of counties were served by both a CCP and a PFFS plan, summing to 17%.) Access to private plans through Medicare has increased substantially since 2004, and now nearly all counties are served by at least one type of private plan, though for half of all counties, PFFS is the only plan type available as of 2008.

Medicare beneficiaries, however, are not equally distributed by counties. This occurs because the population and plans are not distributed equally across counties, but rather they are concentrated in the more urban counties. In 2007, while half of all counties were served by only PFFS plan options, the beneficiaries in those counties represented only 17% of all Medicare beneficiaries (**Table 1**). The proportion of beneficiaries with access limited to PFFS plan options has remained stable since 2001 (prior to the MMA) at between 17% and 20%.

Availability can further be examined taking into account the MA plans set up by employers for their retirees. Though only the retirees of the sponsoring company are eligible to join the plan, their increased popularity in recent years has provided additional options for this subset of Medicare beneficiaries. In 2007, taking into account employer sponsored plans, 96% of all beneficiaries had access to both a coordinated care plan and a private fee for service plan, and 4% of all beneficiaries had access to only a PFFS plan, though again, not all beneficiaries would be eligible to enroll in an employer sponsored plan.

Enrollment Patterns in Urban and Rural Locations

Patterns of Medicare Part C enrollment are not uniform across urban and rural locales, and have varied over time as shown in **Figure 4**. The geographic areas are defined as follows:

- Central urban—central counties of metropolitan areas of at least 1 million population.

- Other urban—either fringe counties of metropolitan areas of at least 1 million population or counties of metropolitan areas up to 1 million population.
- Urban/rural fringe—urban population of at least 2,500 adjacent to a metropolitan area.
- Other rural—includes urban population of at least 2,500, not adjacent to a metropolitan area, and rural areas (defined as places with a population of less than 2,500).

Table 1. Changes in Access to Coordinated Care Plans, Private Fee-for-Service Plans, and Both, by Proportion of Counties and Beneficiaries (selected years 1997 to 2007)

No Existing Plans in County			Managed Care Only		Private Fee-for-Service Only		Both Managed Care and Private Fee-for-Service	
Year	% of counties	% of beneficiaries	% of counties	% of beneficiaries	% of counties	% of beneficiaries	% of counties	% of beneficiaries
1997	76%	NA	24%	NA	0%	NA	0%	NA
1999	71%	NA	29%	NA	0%	NA	0%	NA
2001	37%	18%	10%	43%	43%	18%	10%	21%
2002	38%	21%	10%	43%	44%	18%	8%	18%
2003	37%	21%	9%	42%	46%	20%	8%	17%
2004	31%	16%	13%	42%	44%	19%	12%	23%
2005	4%	2%	4%	21%	53%	18%	39%	58%
2006	1%	1%	3%	18%	54%	19%	42%	62%
2007	0%	0%	0%	0%	50%	17%	50%	82%

Source: MedPAC Computations based on CMS public data for 1997 and 1999; CRS analysis of CMS data for 2003-2003; CMS analysis for 2004-2007.

Notes: NA = not available. The table does not include demonstration plans, cost plans, employer-sponsored plans, regional MA plans, or plans serving Puerto Rico. Medicare managed care includes risk plans through 1998, Medicare+Choice plans through 2003, and Medicare Advantage plans starting in 2004. Managed Care includes the PPO demonstration for 2004 and 2005. Regional MA plans cover 38 or 39 states in 2007, but accounted for less than 2% of enrollment. To determine access to managed care plans regardless of access to PFFS plans, add the percentages for "Managed Care Only" and "Both Managed Care and Private Fee-for-Service." Because of rounding and data technicalities, 100% access or 0 plans are not absolute numbers and should be taken as accurate approximations.

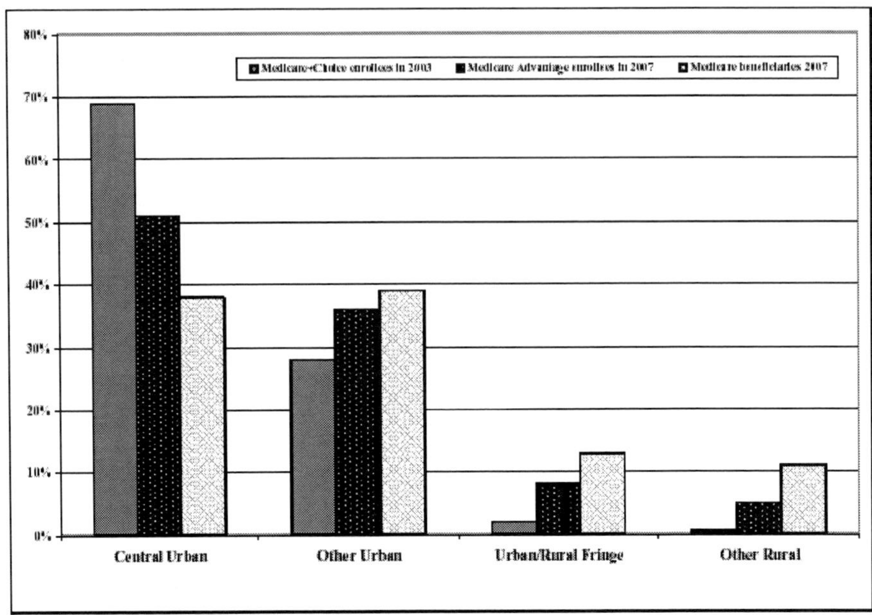

Source: Prepared by CRS based on CMS data.

Figure 4. Concentration of Medicare Beneficiaries (2007), Medicare Advantage Enrollees (2007), and Medicare+Choice Enrollees (2003) in Urban and Rural Locations

In 2003, most M+C enrollees resided in central urban areas; about 69% of the M+C population lived in a central urban area in 2003. This percentage decreased to 51% in 2007. However, a smaller proportion, only 39% of all Medicare beneficiaries reside in the central urban areas. (The urban and rural pattern of beneficiary residence as defined above remained the same from 2003 to 2007.) In all geographic areas, except central urban areas, the percentages enrolled in private plans are less than the percentage of Medicare beneficiaries overall. (For example, 13% of Medicare beneficiaries live in the urban/rural fringe areas, but MA enrollees in those areas made up only 8% of total private plan enrollment in 2007, up from 2% of private plan enrollment in 2003.) This means that a larger proportion of the Medicare population in the central urban areas choose to enroll in Medicare private plans relative to other geographic areas; conversely, a lower proportion of beneficiaries choose to enroll in private plans in non-central urban areas, though that trend is decreasing.

Historically, the high enrollment trend in central urban areas occurred because of a combination of interrelated factors, such as historic patterns of managed care enrollment in the non-Medicare market, availability of different plans, and plan benefits. More recently, with greater availability of private plans in suburban and rural areas, more beneficiaries living in those areas are enrolling in MA plans; the urban concentration of MA enrollment is decreasing.

Regional and Geographic Variation in Enrollment

In addition to rural and urban variations, enrollment patterns also vary on a regional basis, though not by as much as in previous years. MA enrollment is slightly higher in western and southwestern states, as shown in **Figure 5**. Approximately 36% of the beneficiaries in Arizona, 34% of the beneficiaries in California, and 38% of the beneficiaries in Oregon are in MA plans. The highest levels of enrollment in the eastern states are in Rhode Island (35%), Florida (26%), Pennsylvania (33%), and New York (25%). Only one state, Alaska, has less than 1% of beneficiaries enrolled in MA. Seventeen states have enrollment of 10% or less. A total of 34 states have enrollment of less than the national average of 21%.

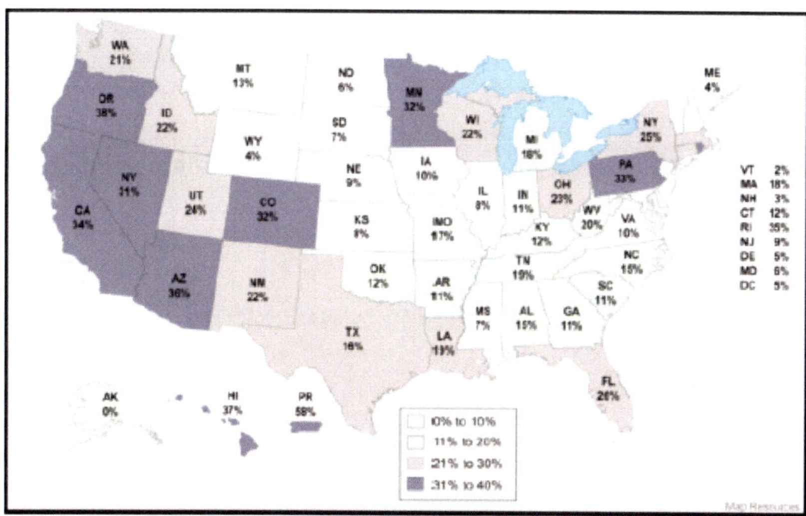

Source: Prepared by CRS based on data from the Centers for Medicare and Medicaid Services.

Notes: State numbers represent percentages.

Figure 5. Percentage of Medicare Beneficiaries Enrolled in Medicare Advantage, by State, January 2008

Table 2. Shares of Medicare+Choice and Medicare Advantage Enrollment and Medicare Population Residing in Four States (January 2003 and 2008)

State	% of Total Medicare Population	% of Total M+C Population in 2003	% of Total MA Enrollment in 2008
California	10	28	16
Florida	7	12	9
Pennsylvania	5	10	8
New York	7	9	8
Total	30	59	41

Source: Prepared by CRS based on data from CMS.

Notes: Numbers may not add due to rounding. Proportion of total Medicare population in each state remained the same from 2003 to 2008.

MA enrollees are more concentrated geographically than Medicare beneficiaries as a whole, though this trend has decreased from 2003 to 2008. In 2003, the four states with the highest percentage of beneficiaries enrolled in Medicare Part C accounted for over half of all enrollment: California, Florida, Pennsylvania, and New York. These four states accounted for 59% of all enrollees in 2003, but they are home to only 30 % of all Medicare beneficiaries. In 2007, enrollment has become slightly less concentrated, with enrollment in those four states accounting for 41% of all MA enrollment. **Table 2** compares the percent of Medicare Part C enrollment to the percent of the total Medicare population for each of these four states.

RULES FOR ELIGIBILITY AND ENROLLMENT

The MA program includes specific rules regarding eligibility to enroll in a private plan, and when enrollment can take place. The following is a description of those requirements.

Eligibility

Medicare beneficiaries are eligible to enroll in any MA plan that serves their area, with the following restrictions: (1) beneficiaries must be entitled to benefits under Part A of Medicare and enrolled in Part B of Medicare and (2) beneficiaries who qualify for Medicare solely on the basis of end-stage renal disease (ESRD) may not enroll in an MA plan. Three exceptions apply to individuals with ESRD: (1) a beneficiary enrolled in an MA plan who later develops ESRD may continue to remain enrolled in that plan; (2) if a plan terminates its contract or reduces its service area (for an enrollee this is referred to as an involuntary termination), ESRD enrollees may enroll in another MA plan; and (3) an individual with ESRD may elect to enroll in an MA SNP as long as the plan has opted to enroll ESRD individuals. Members of an Employer Group Health Plan (EGHP) may also elect their employer's MA plan even if the individual resides outside the MA plan service area provided the plan meets certain access requirements.

Residency Requirements

An MA eligible individual may only enroll in an MA plan that serves the geographic area in which the individual resides, with two exceptions: (1) a plan may allow an individual to remain in a local plan, even if he or she no longer resides in the service area, so long as the plan provides reasonable access within that geographic area to the full range of basic benefits, with reasonable cost sharing, and (2) a local MA organization that eliminates a payment area previously within its service area may choose to offer enrollees in all or part of the affected area continued enrollment in the plan, under certain conditions. Local HMOs may determine their own service area, consisting of counties or equivalent areas. Nothing prevents a local plan from being offered in more than one MA area.

Enrollment Periods

In general, MA organizations can enroll Medicare eligible individuals during four enrollment periods: (1) initial coverage election period, (2) annual election period, (3) open enrollment period, and (4) special election periods. The initial coverage election period applies to newly eligible Medicare beneficiaries, who are allowed to enroll in an MA plan up to three months prior to their Medicare entitlement date. During the annual coordinated election period (November 15-December 31), all MA eligible beneficiaries can enroll or disenroll from any MA plan, or switch from original Medicare to MA, or MA to original Medicare. Changes in elections are made during the open enrollment period. The open enrollment period allows individuals to make one change during the first three months of the year. Beneficiaries in original Medicare can enroll in an MA plan, and individuals enrolled in an MA plan can either switch to a different MA plan or return to original Medicare. However, during the three-month open enrollment period, beneficiaries cannot change their drug coverage. For example, an individual enrolled in a MA-PD plan can elect only to enroll in another MA-PD plan. Similarly, an individual enrolled in original Medicare and a stand-alone PDP can change only to an MA-PD plan. The reverse is true as well.

Individuals enrolled in original Medicare without drug coverage can enroll only in MA plans that do not offer drug coverage. Eligible beneficiaries who are institutionalized may change their election any time during the year.

Special Election Periods

Outside the annual coordinated election period and open election period, beneficiaries can change their enrollment status only under special circumstances, called Special Election Periods (SEPs). The Secretary has created SEPs for the following instances: (1) when the organization has terminated its contract or discontinued offering its plan in the resident's service area, (2) the resident moves to a new service area, (3) the beneficiary can demonstrate that the plan has violated the terms of its contract (i.e., fails to provide medically necessary care or misrepresents the plan in its marketing materials), or (4) the individual meets other exceptional circumstances provided by CMS.

SUPPLEMENTAL BENEFITS

Nearly all plans offer some benefits to enrollees beyond those in original Medicare. All supplemental benefits are paid for either with (1) a rebate earned by the plan through the bidding process, (2) directly by the enrollee through a supplemental premium, or (3) some combination of a plan rebate and supplemental premium. A Government Accountability Office (GAO) analysis of MA plan supplemental benefits (as projected by the plans in their 2007 bid documents) indicated that, overall, rebates paid for 77% of supplemental benefits, and additional premiums paid for the remaining 23%. However, the proportions varied by plan. Other analyses have examined supplemental benefits offered to enrollees in the lowest premium package offered by each participating organization; benefits in these packages would be more likely to be paid for through savings rather than a supplemental premium. These analyses found that in 2005, most MA enrollees were offered vision care (92%) and hearing coverage (99%), while all were offered routine physicals (100%) (**Figure 6**). Prescription drug coverage was a popular supplemental benefit prior to the start of the new Medicare Part D prescription drug program; with the Part D program, some type of prescription drug coverage is available to all enrollees who choose to join an MA plan that covers drugs. **Figure 6** shows that the percentage of enrollees offered these benefits has fluctuated for all services between 1999 and 2005. However, the figure does not show how the extent of benefits or the level of cost sharing may have changed over the time period

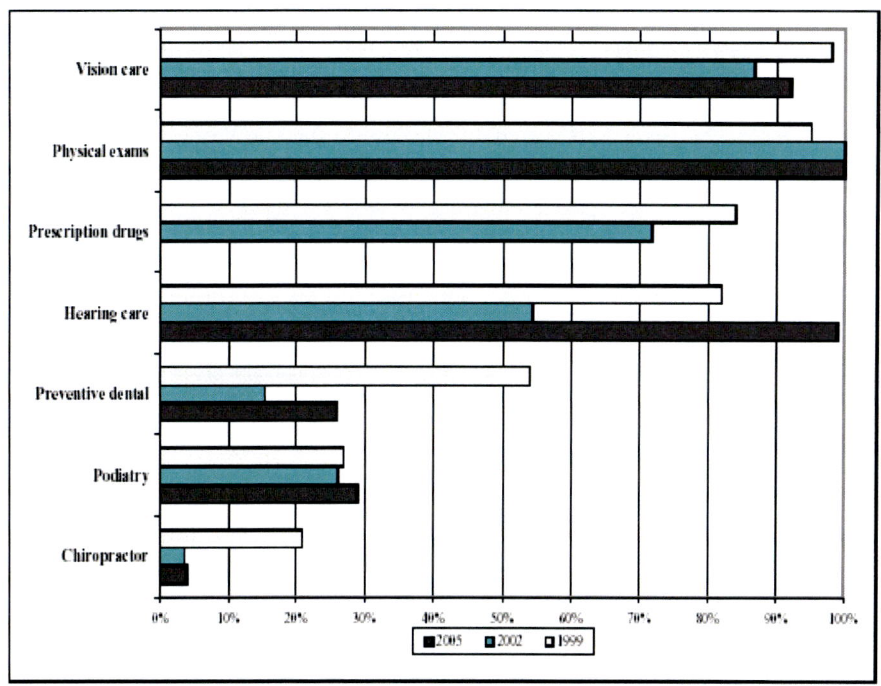

Source: Chart prepared by CRS based on Mathematica Policy Research analysis of CMS data.

Figure 6. Percentage of M+C and M.A. Enrollees Offered Benefits Beyond Traditional Medicare Covered Services, in the Lowest Premium Padage Available, 1999, 2002, and 2005

PREMIUMS

All MA enrollees are required to pay the Part B premium, although plans may pay this for their enrollees as a supplemental benefit. Plans are permitted to charge enrollees additional out-of-pocket fees, such as premiums and coinsurance, depending on which plan the individual elects. Any supplemental premium charged to plan enrollees is a consolidation of any of the following three charges: (1) a premium to cover basic Part A and B benefits if a plan bid was above the benchmark, (2) a premium to cover supplemental benefits not paid for through a plan rebate, and (3) a premium for Part D prescription drug coverage. However, plans have an incentive to minimize supplemental premiums in order to remain competitive in local markets.

Between 1999 and 2003, the percentage of beneficiaries nationally with access to a zero premium coordinated care plan declined. As shown in **Table 3**, the availability of these plans dropped by half, from over 60% to just under 30%. Between 2003 and 2006, access to a zero premium plan doubled, again achieving the previous high of 61%. The percentage of beneficiaries enrolled in a zero premium coordinated care plan has fluctuated as well, but changes in the methodology make a comparison of this measure over time difficult. In 2006, just over half of MA coordinated care plan enrollees were in a plan with a zero combined premium for Part C and Part D benefits.

COVERAGE FOR PRESCRIPTION DRUGS

Prior to 2006, one of the advantages of Medicare private plans over original Medicare was that most plans included some outpatient prescription drug coverage. The MMA added the Medicare Part D prescription drug program, making some type of drug coverage available to all beneficiaries. With one exception, every MA organization in an area is required to offer at least one Medicare Advantage-Prescription Drug (MA-PD) plan, one that offers qualified Part D prescription drug coverage. PFFS plans are not required to offer a plan with qualified prescription drug benefits. If a beneficiary enrolls in a PFFS plan that does not provide prescription drug coverage, he or she can enroll in a stand-alone Part D prescription drug plan in addition to the PFFS plan. Beneficiaries who choose any other MA plan without drug coverage can not enroll in a stand alone Part D plan.

Table 3. Changes in Access to or Coverage Under a Medicare+Choice or Medicare Advantage Coordinated Care Plan with a Zero Premium, 1999 to 2006

Year	Overall Medicare Population with Access to Zero Premium Coordinated Care Plan	Enrollees with Zero Premium Coordinated Care Plan
1999	61	68
2000	53	61
2001	39	45
2002	34	39
2003	29	38
2004	40	48[a]
2005	42	58[a]
2006	61	52[b]

Source: Centers for Medicare and Medicaid Services. Analysis of submitted bids from Health Plan Management System (HPMS) data; data development by the Office of Research, Development and Information.

Notes: This table does not include Private Fee-or-Service or employer sponsored plans. It includes Special Needs Plans, Health maintenance Organizations, Preferred Provider Organizations, and Provider Sponsored Organizations.

a. Enrollment in zero premium plan reflects actual enrollment as reported by the plan. In prior years, enrollees were assigned to the zero premium plan if one was available.

b. For 2006, zero premium refers to the combined part C and part D premium.

MA organizations offering prescription drug coverage receive a direct subsidy for each enrollee in an MA-PD plan equal to the plan's adjusted standardized bid amount for its prescription drug benefit (reduced by the base beneficiary Part D premium). The plan also receives the reinsurance payment amount of 80% of the costs for drugs exceeding the annual out-of-pocket threshold for an enrollee ($4,050 in 2008). Finally, MA-PD plans receive reimbursement for premium cost- sharing reductions for their qualifying low-income enrollees.

Beneficiaries who enroll in an MA plan offering Part D must pay the plan the standard Part D premium. However, MA-PD plans that receive a rebate in the bidding process may use all or part of that rebate as a credit toward the MA monthly prescription drug premium.

Beneficiary Protections

The MA program includes requirements designed to limit beneficiaries' financial liability and to assure beneficiaries of certain rights. Among these beneficiary protections are standards to ensure access to Medicare benefits and providers, beneficiary liability standards, health care quality standards, consumer disclosure and plan marketing requirements, and a grievance and appeals process.

Enrollment

In general, MA organizations cannot deny enrollment on the basis of health status-related factors. These factors include health status, medical condition (including both physical and mental illnesses), claims experience, receipt of health care, medical history, genetic information, evidence of insurability (including conditions arising out of acts of domestic violence), and disability. However, an organization may deny enrollment if it has reached the limits of its capacity. Organizations may terminate an enrollee's election only for failure to pay premiums on a timely basis, disruptive behavior, or because the plan ends for all MA enrollees.

Access to Providers

Coordinated care plans such as HMOs and PPOs are required to form provider networks to meet Medicare access requirements. In accordance with network requirements, each provider has a written contract or agreement to furnish services to plan enrollees. Care is generally not covered or is partially covered if received from a provider who is not in the plan's network. Regional PPOs, despite being coordinated care plans, can use methods other than written agreements to meet access requirements with the Secretary's approval.

Prior to 2011, however, PFFS plans are not required to establish networks of providers. PFFS plans must permit enrollees to obtain services from any Medicare participating provider that agrees to the plans' terms and conditions. PFFS plans meet access requirements by (1) establishing payment rates that are not less than those under original FFS Medicare or (2) having signed (direct) contracts with a sufficient number and range of providers in a particular category. Most PFFS plans are meeting access requirements by paying providers the same rates as original Medicare. Starting in 2011, PFFS plans sponsored by employers or unions are required to establish contracted networks of providers to meet access requirements. Non-employer-sponsored MA PFFS plans are required to establish contracted networks of providers in network areas defined as areas having at least two plans with networks (such as HMOs, PSOs, or local PPOs). In areas without at least two network based plans, the non-employer PFFS plans retain the ability to establish access requirements through establishing payment rates that are not less than those under original Medicare.

Enrollees in PFFS plans may obtain covered services from any Medicare eligible provider who is willing to furnish services and accepts the plan's terms and conditions of participation. However, the lack of a written agreement between the plan and provider (in areas where PFFS plans do not have a contracted network of providers) means that the providers are not required to treat plan enrollees. Providers may determine on a case-by-case or visit-by-visit basis whether to serve a plan's enrollees.

Other access requirements include developing written standards to ensure that access to care is timely; developing policies and procedures in the areas of coverage, payment, and utilization; and establishing written requirements for ensuring beneficiary input in a treatment plan. Plans must also ensure that services are available 24 hours a day 7 days a week and provide access to ambulance and emergency services.

Access to Benefits

CMS reviews and approves MA plan benefit offerings, including mandatory and optional supplemental benefits, to ensure that plans are providing all Part A and B covered services (except hospice), do not discriminate against beneficiaries, do not discourage enrollment or encourage disenrollment, do not steer subsets of Medicare beneficiaries to certain MA plans, or inhibit access to services. CMS also reviews mandatory supplemental benefits (i.e., benefits not covered under original Medicare, reduced Medicare premiums, or cost-sharing amounts) to ensure that they are designed in accordance with CMS's guidelines and requirements.

Beneficiary Financial Liability Protections

Enrollees in MA-coordinated care plans (i.e., HMOs and PPOs) are likely to experience the least amount of out-of-pocket costs (compared to other MA plans). Cost sharing per enrollee (excluding premiums) for covered services cannot be more than the actuarial value of the deductibles, coinsurance, and co-payments under traditional Medicare. However, while the aggregate amount of cost sharing in an MA plan must be equal to the aggregate amount of cost sharing in original Medicare, the plan may set different amounts for specific services, such as a lower (or higher) deductible for hospital inpatient services or skilled nursing facility services.

Balance billing under Medicare generally refers to an amount billed by a provider in excess of Medicare's recognized payment amount (which includes beneficiary cost sharing). Original Medicare prohibits balance billing by Medicare-"participating physicians" but allows nonparticipating physicians to balance bill up to 115% of the non-participating Medicare fee- schedule amount, which is 9.25% above the recognized amount for participating providers.

Providers participating in coordinated care MA plans, such as HMOs, are prohibited from balance billing. However, providers participating in PFFS plans are allowed to balance bill enrollees up to 115% of the plan's fee schedule, subject to the terms and conditions of the plan. This means that if a PFFS plan allows providers to balance bill, the beneficiary would be responsible for any balance billing charges in addition to any cost-sharing required by the plan. If the PFFS plan does not allow balance billing, the beneficiary is not responsible for balance billing charges, but would be responsible for any cost-sharing requirements under the plan. Balance billing rules under PFFS plans may apply to all types of Medicare providers. PFFS plans are obliged to inform beneficiaries of these balance billing amounts, and hospitals are required to provide PFFS enrollees advanced notice of balance billing charges.

Quality Standards

All MA organizations are required to have a quality improvement program. As part of the quality improvement program, plans must collect, analyze, and report data to measure health outcomes and other indices. Specific requirements include designing a chronic care improvement program, conducting quality improvement projects, and encouraging providers to participate in CMS and HHS quality initiatives. Plans are required to annually assess the impact and effectiveness of their quality improvement programs and take timely action to correct any systemic problems that come to their attention.

CMS requires that MA plans collect and report on a subset of performance measures from the National Committee for Quality Assurance's (NCQA's) Health Plan Employer Data and Information Set (HEDIS), the Consumer Assessment of Health Plans Study (CAHPS), and the Medicare Health Outcomes Survey (HOS).

Consumer Disclosure Requirements

MA organizations must disclose to each enrollee (at the time of enrollment and at least annually) information on their service area, benefits, the number, mix, and distribution of providers, out-ofarea coverage, emergency coverage, supplemental benefits, prior authorization rules, plan grievance and appeals procedures, the quality improvement program, disenrollment rights and responsibilities, and cost-sharing obligations. MA organizations must make a good faith effort to provide enrollees with written notice of a provider's termination from the plan's network at least 30 days prior to the termination date. Medicare-eligible enrollees are also allowed to request from the plan information on procedures used by the organization to control utilization, the number of grievances and appeals, a description of physician compensation practices, and descriptions of the plan's financial performance. When an MA organization terminates its contract with CMS, it must provide and pay for advance written notice to each of its enrollees, along with a description of alternatives for obtaining benefits.

Marketing Requirements

MA organizations are required to submit marketing brochures and enrollment forms to CMS for review and approval at least 45 days before distribution. If using CMS model materials, the approval time is reduced from 45 to 10 days. As part of the review process, CMS must ensure that the information provided to beneficiaries is not inaccurate or misleading. MA organizations are also required to develop marketing materials that provide an adequate description of plan benefits, providers, and fees; an explanation of the grievance and appeals process; notification of the open enrollment period; and a statement indicating that either the plan or CMS can terminate the contract, thereby resulting in the beneficiary's disenrollment from the plan.

CMS has also developed standards for regulating the marketing conduct of MA organizations. These standards include prohibitions against door-to-door soliciting, providing cash or other monetary rebates to induce enrollment, and conducting misleading or confusing activities, such as claiming that the MA organization has been endorsed by CMS or Medicare. Further, providers cannot distribute information to beneficiaries comparing benefits across plans or allow beneficiaries to complete enrollment applications in provider offices.

CMS issued a proposed rule in May 2008 changing some marketing standards into regulations. Prior to the issuance of a final rule, MIPPA established the following new prohibitions on the marketing activities of MA plans. Except in instances where the beneficiary initiates contact, plans will be prohibited from soliciting beneficiaries door-to-door or on the phone. Cross-selling of non-health products, providing meals to prospective enrollees, marketing or selling plans at educational events or in areas where health care is delivered (i.e., physician offices or pharmacies), and using sales agents that are not state licensed are also prohibited. MIPPA required that by November 15, 2008, the Secretary establish limitations on other plan marketing activities such as co-branding, the scope of marketing appointments with prospective enrollees, and agent compensation and training. MA plans will be required to provide states with information on (1) agent and broker terminations and (2) at state request, performance and licensing of agents, brokers, and any third party representing the plan. After January 1, 2010, MA plans will be required to include the plan type in all plan names. Some provisions included in the CMS proposed rule were not included in MIPPA but may be addressed in the final rule, including (1) a requirement that, upon CMS's request, MA plans would be required to provide any information necessary to conduct oversight of marketing activities, and (2) development of a memorandum of understanding between states and CMS to share compliance and oversight information.

Grievance and Appeals

An MA organization must have procedures for hearing and resolving grievances between the organization and enrollees. It also must maintain a process for making timely organization determinations, which are plan decisions related to enrollees' benefits and payment. Beneficiaries have 60 days from the date of service to file a grievance with their MA plan. Beneficiaries have the right to a timely resolution to their grievance (no later than 30 days) as well as the right to request an appeal or reconsideration of an organization determination. In certain circumstances, beneficiaries may also request an expedited determination, which requires a decision be rendered in 72 hours. All MA organizations are required to provide written information to enrollees about these processes. They are also required to inform beneficiaries about how to initiate quality of care complaints to their local Quality Improvement Organization (QIO). The QIO complaint process is distinct from the MA organization's grievance procedure, and beneficiaries have the right to file a complaint with the MA organization and QIO simultaneously. All quality-of-care complaints and adverse organization determinations must be responded to in writing.

PROGRAM STANDARDS AND CONTRACT REQUIREMENTS

The MA program requires the private health plans that participate to meet minimum program standards and contracting requirements. These requirements include minimum enrollment standards, organizational and financial requirements as specified by states, provider protections, and prompt payment requirements. The Secretary is required to conduct audits of at least one- third of MA participating organizations each year. In the event that organizations violate the standards and requirements, the Secretary had the authority to terminate the contract or impose sanctions.

Minimum Enrollment Standards

Contracts between MA organizations and CMS are made for at least one year and are automatically renewable, unless either party gives notice to terminate the contract. MA organizations must enroll at least 5,000 individuals (1,500 in the case of a PSO) or at least 1,500 individuals (500 in the case of a PSO) if the organization serves individuals residing outside of urbanized areas. These minimum requirements may be waived during the first three years of the contract, if the organization can demonstrate to CMS that it can administer and manage an MA contract and also manage the level of risk required under the contract.

Organizational and Financial Requirements

In general, an MA organization must be licensed under state law as a risk-bearing entity eligible to offer health insurance or health benefits coverage in each state in which it offers an MA plan. An MA organization must assume full risk for Medicare benefits on a prospective basis. However, this does not preclude an organization from obtaining insurance or making other arrangements to cover certain costs, such as medically necessary services provided by non-network providers and part of the costs exceeding its income. The organization also may make arrangements with providers to assume some or all of the financial risk for covered benefits they provide; however, PFFS organizations cannot put providers at risk.

Provider Protections and Requirements

Each MA organization (other than a PFFS) must establish physician participation procedures that provide (1) notice of the participation rules, (2) written notice of adverse participation decisions, and (3) a process for appealing adverse decisions. The organization must consult with contracting physicians regarding the organization's medical policy, quality, and medical management procedures.

Although plans may include providers only to the extent necessary to meet the needs of their enrollees, they cannot discriminate with respect to providers who are acting within the scope of their license or certification under applicable state law, solely on the basis of such license or certification. Restricting communications between providers and their patients (a gag clause) is prohibited. The use of physician financial incentive plans, (compensation arrangements between organizations and individual or groups of physicians that may reduce or limit services) is also limited.

Protections Against Fraud

The Secretary is required to conduct annual audits of the financial records of at least one-third of the MA participating organizations (including data relating to utilization, costs, and computation of the plan's bid). The Secretary also has the right to inspect and audit the quality, appropriateness, and timeliness of the services provided to enrollees, as well as any records pertaining to the organization's ability to bear risk. In addition, HHS, GAO, or their designee has the right to audit and evaluate an MA organization's records and those of its subcontractors that pertain to the services provided under the contract. This right extends for 10 years from the termination date of the final contract. If CMS suspects potential fraud, the agency may conduct an inspection or audit of the MA organization at any time.

Prompt Payment Requirements

MA PFFS plans are required to pay 95% of "clean claims" within 30 days of receipt. This 30-day rule also applies to claims submitted to any MA organization by a provider who does not have a written contact with the plan. MA organizations are required to pay interest on "clean claims" that are not paid within 30 days. All other claims from non-contracted providers must be paid within 60 days. MA organizations that do contract with providers (i.e., HMOs and PPOs) must include a prompt payment provision in their contracts. CMS defines a clean claim as a claim that has no defect or impropriety, and is submitted with all the required documentation.

Contract Terminations and Sanctions

The Secretary has the authority to terminate an annual contract with an MA plan if the MA organization fails substantially to carry out the terms of its contract. Reasons for termination can be severe financial difficulties, failing to comply with required grievance and appeals procedures, failing to implement an acceptable quality assessment and performance improvement program, failing to comply with CMS marketing requirements, and committing fraud. Except in instances where the MA organization is experiencing severe financial hardship, CMS is required to provide the organization with an opportunity to develop a corrective action plan (CAP) to correct any deficiencies before terminating the contract. MA organizations have the right to appeal a termination. MA organizations also have the right to terminate their contract with CMS if CMS fails to substantially carry out the terms of its contract.

The Secretary has the authority to impose sanctions, including civil monetary penalties, on MA organizations in the following eight instances: (1) failing to provide medically necessary services, which result in an adverse outcome for the patient; (2) charging excess beneficiary premiums; (3) expelling or refusing to reenroll individuals in violation of stated requirements; (4) denying or discouraging enrollment of individuals whose medical condition requires future services; (5) misrepresenting or falsifying information to the Secretary or others; (6) interfering with practitioners advice to enrollees; (7) failing to comply with rules regarding physician participation and balance billing; and (8) contracting with excluded providers. In addition to civil monetary penalties, the Secretary can temporarily suspend enrollment in the plan, stop payment, and restrict the MA organization's marketing activities. The civil monetary penalties may range from $10,000 to $100,000, depending on the nature of the violation.

ISSUES FOR CONGRESS

The 111th Congress may examine several aspects of the Medicare Advantage program, including the difference in expenditures per beneficiary between MA and original Medicare, profits reported by MA plans, the Comparative Cost Adjustment Program mandated under the MMA, and marketing issues.

Per Beneficiary Expenditure Differences between MA and Original Medicare

Medicare-managed care plans may have the potential to provide better quality care at less cost than original Medicare.[5] In fact, prior to the BBA, private plans were paid 95% of the cost of Medicare, in part because of this presumed greater efficiency. However, the current payment mechanism does not encourage plans to be more efficient than original Medicare, because it pays plans at least as much as the cost of Medicare, and on average, more. According to the Medicare Payment Advisory Commission (MedPac), Medicare is expected to pay private plans an average of 14% more per beneficiary in 2009 than it does for beneficiaries enrolled in the original Medicare program. In 2008, the *maximum* amount Medicare was willing to pay MA plans to provide Medicare covered benefits was, on average, 18% higher than the estimated cost of providing those same benefits under original Medicare.[6] MA health maintenance organizations were the only plan type that, on average, estimated their cost of providing Medicare-covered benefits at below the cost of original Medicare; this suggests MA health maintenance organizations can be more cost effective than original Medicare.

MA plans use at least part of the payments (above the cost of original Medicare) to provide extra benefits and reduced cost sharing to enrollees. In addition, these higher payments have attracted private plans to areas previously underserved by Medicare private plans, and beneficiaries today have more private plans to choose from than they did 10 years ago. However, the higher payments (1) allow inefficient plans to continue participating in Medicare, (2) contribute to the financial instability of the program in the long-run, and (3) increase Part B premium costs for all beneficiaries in the Medicare program. Moreover, the reported quality data for MA plans are limited and variable.[7] Both MA payments and quality measures are to be addressed in upcoming MedPac reports to Congress.[8] Specifically, MedPac is to study how comparable measures of performance and patient experience can be collected and reported by 2011 for MA and original Medicare. The second study requires MedPac to study the relationship between plan bids and per capita spending in original Medicare, alternatives to county level payments, and the accuracy and completeness of county-level spending estimates.

Congress may choose to reexamine MA payments and whether the amount paid to MA plans above the cost of original Medicare should remain part of the MA payment, or whether that money should be used for other priorities. If Congress chooses to reduce spending in the MA program, there are many different ways of achieving these savings. Reducing payments, regardless of the method, may result in reduced supplemental benefits or reduced access to plans. However, each individual option would have different pros and cons.

One provision included in the House-passed H.R. 3162, the Children's Health and Medicare Protection (CHAMP) Act of 2007, would have phased in MA benchmarks equal to per capita feefor-service (FFS) spending in each county, effectively decreasing MA benchmarks in all areas where it exceeded average Medicare spending. MA plans would need to be as efficient as original Medicare in order to continue serving Medicare beneficiaries. This provision was not taken up by the Senate. The Congressional Budget Office (CBO) estimated that setting benchmarks equal to spending in original Medicare could save $55 billion over 5 years and $157 billion over 10 years.[9] Though this method would eliminate the unequal expenditures between MA and original Medicare—sometimes referred to as "creating a level playing field"—it could result in decreased access to MA plans in rural and some urban areas, thus increasing a geographic difference that was prevalent through all but the most recent years of the program.

Other options would reduce payments while allowing for some differences between MA and original Medicare. Some argue that certain costs faced by private plans, such as administrative costs and payments to health care providers, are not the same as those of original Medicare, and therefore, the maximum amount Medicare pays private plans should not be as low as original Medicare in some areas.[10] In such case, benchmarks could take into account the estimated costs of MA plans, much like the Regional MA plans. The CBO estimated that basing benchmarks on plan bids could save $35 billion over 5 years and $158 billion over 10 years.[11] This option would not create a level playing field between MA and original Medicare. However, it would still achieve some savings and might not have as severe an effect on access to plans, as the cost to plans of serving a particular area would be used to calculate the benchmark for the area.

Another option would be an across-the-board percentage cut in benchmarks. In higher benchmark areas where the benchmark is more likely based on per capita FFS spending, the reduction may resemble the payment policy prior to the BBA when plans were paid a percentage of spending in original Medicare. Depending on the size of the reduction, it is possible that benchmarks for many rural and some urban areas would remain above spending in original Medicare. Again, this option would not create a level playing field between MA and original Medicare. Another disadvantage is that it does not incorporate information from the plans to gauge the cost of doing business in a particular market. However, the largest reductions would occur in high payment rate areas where some of the tools of managed care, such as establishing provider networks and coordinating patient care, may be easier to employ.

Medical Expenditures and Profits

Other issues have arisen with respect to MA plan payments. Recent congressional attention has focused on the profits earned by MA plans. Two analyses by the Government Accountability Office found that MA organizations generally spent less on providing medical services than the plans had estimated they would.[12] As a result, the profit margins for these plans was higher, on average, than plans had predicted. These findings held for 2005 and 2006, resulting in over $1 billion in additional profits to MA plans each year. The 111th Congress may opt to consider whether to limit MA plan profits in an effort to either reduce overall Medicare spending, or to increase the extra benefits and reduced cost sharing these plans offer to enrollees.

The House-passed CHAMP Act of 2007 included a provision that would have required the Secretary to publish the percentage of plan revenues that were spent on clinical services, as distinct from administration and profit. This amount is often referred to as the Medical Loss Ratio (MLR).[13] The bill also required plans with MLRs below a specified level to face reduced benchmarks, limited enrollment, and possible termination. These provisions in CHAMP were not taken up in the Senate.

Comparative Cost Adjustment in 2010

Beginning in 2010, the Secretary will establish a program for the application of comparative cost adjustment (CCA) in CCA areas. The six-year program will begin January 1, 2010, and end December 31, 2015. The program is designed to test direct competition among local MA plans, as well as competition between local MA plans and fee-for-service Medicare. This program will occur only in a limited number of statutorily qualifying areas in the country.

The benchmark for MA local plans in a CCA area will be calculated using a formula that weights (1) the projected FFS spending in an area (with certain adjustments for demographics and health status) and (2) a weighted average of plan bids.

For Medicare beneficiaries in traditional Medicare, Part B premiums in CCA areas will be adjusted either up or down, depending on whether the FFS amount is more or less than the CCA area benchmark. If the FFS amount is greater than the benchmark, beneficiaries in traditional Medicare FFS will pay a higher Part B premium than other FFS beneficiaries in non-CCA areas. If the FFS amount is less than the benchmark, the Part B premium for FFS beneficiaries will be reduced by 75% of the difference. These increases and decreases are subject to a 5% limit; that is, adjustments to Part B premiums in CCA areas cannot exceed 5% of the national part B premium. Beneficiaries in traditional Medicare FFS with incomes below 150% of poverty, who qualify for low-income subsidies under the Medicare prescription drug program, will not have their Part B premium increased.

In the 110th Congress, the House passed legislation to repeal the CCA demonstration, but that provision was not taken up by the Senate. Historically, potential cost saving programs have generated opposition resulting in delays or cancellations.[14] Generally, Members have not supported demonstrations or programs that have the potential to adversely affect companies or beneficiaries in their districts. The Secretary has not announced the locations of the CCA demonstrations.

Marketing

Questionable marketing practices by MA plans, their agents, or brokers has attracted congressional attention. During the 110th Congress, several committees held hearings identifying the allegedly deceptive and aggressive sales practices of some MA plans, such as door-to-door solicitations, misleading beneficiaries about plan coverage, and signing beneficiaries up for a plan without their knowledge. Hearings also investigated factors that may have encouraged aggressive marketing practices, such as the structure of agent and broker compensation. Though many of the behaviors identified in the hearings were prohibited by CMS guidance, they were not explicitly prohibited by statutes or regulations. On May 16, 2008, CMS issued a proposed rule to codify into regulations some of the marketing policies already in the marketing guidance. Following the proposed rule, Congress passed the Medicare Improvements for Patients and Providers Act of 2008 (MIPPA, P.L. 110-275), which codified into statutes some of the provisions in the proposed rule, including (1) prohibiting door-to-door solicitations and other agent-initiated contact; (2) clarifying that sales activities are only permitted in common areas of health care settings and prohibited in areas primarily used for patient care; (3) prohibiting sales activities (such as distribution of applications) at educational events; and (4) requiring that MA and Part D plans only use state-licensed, certified, or registered marketing representatives in states that require using such agents. MIPPA also directed the Secretary to establish guidelines on agent commissions to ensure that commissions encouraged agents to enroll beneficiaries in plans that best met their health care needs. A revised interim final rule established compensation levels for agents and brokers based on historical compensation levels in the same market, adjusted for whether or not this was the first year the beneficiary had enrolled in a particular plan type. Compensation would be decreased if the beneficiary disenrolled from the plan within the first year. It is unclear whether marketing issues for Medicare private plans will garner congressional attention going in the 111th congress. While it appears that the legislation resolved many of the issues, Congress will have to wait and see whether or not those conducting the abusive practices are able to circumvent the changes to the law.

APPENDIX. LEGISLATIVE HISTORY, 1997 TO 2008

This section summarizes major legislation enacted into law that modifies Medicare Part C, beginning in 1997. The summary highlights major provisions; it is not a comprehensive list of all Medicare amendments. Included are provisions that had a significant budget impact, changed program benefits, modified beneficiary cost sharing, or involved major program reforms. Provisions involving policy changes are mentioned the first time they are incorporated in legislation, but not necessarily every time a modification is made. The descriptions include either the initial effective date of the provision or, in the case of budget savings provisions, the fiscal years for which cuts were specified.

Balanced Budget Act of 1997 (BBA, P.L. 105-33)

The BBA established a new part C of Medicare called Medicare+Choice (M+C). It was built on the existing Medicare Risk Contract Program, which enabled beneficiaries to enroll, where available, in health maintenance organizations (HMOs) that contracted with the Medicare Program. It expanded, beginning in 1999, the private plan options that could contract with Medicare to other types of private health care organizations (e.g., PPOs and PSOs), PFFS, and, on a limited demonstration basis, high deductible plans (called MSA plans) offered in conjunction with savings accounts.

Prior to BBA, the payment for private plans was based on 95% of the average adjusted per capita cost (AAPCC) of beneficiaries in original Medicare in each county. BBA replaced that payment methodology with a formula that calculated the highest of three amounts calculated *for each county*: (1) a blended rate, which was blend of an area-specific (local) rate and a national rate; (2) a minimum payment (or floor) rate; or (3) a rate reflecting a minimum increase from the previous year's rate. Payment rates under this formula were subject to a budget neutrality provision such that the total amount of payments under the formula methodology could not be greater or less than the payments in the absence of the formula. The blended per capita rate was intended to shift payment amounts away from local (generally county) rates, which reflected the wide variations in fee-for-service costs, toward a national average rate. The floor rate was designed to raise payments in certain counties more quickly than would occur through the blend alone, and the minimum increase percentage was to protect counties that would otherwise receive only a small (if any) increase.

BBA established an M+C Competitive Pricing Demonstration Project in seven payment areas. Under the demonstration, payments to M+C organizations would be determined competitively, as determined by the Secretary in consultation with an advisory committee.

Balanced Budget Refinement Act of 1999 (BBRA, P.L. 106-113)

BBRA contained several provisions designed to facilitate the implementation of M+C. It changed the phase-in of the new risk adjustment payment methodology based on health status to a blend of 10% new health status method/90% old demographic method in 2000 and 2001, and not more than 20% health status in 2002. It provided for payment of a new entry bonus of 5% of the monthly M+C payment rate in the first 12 months and 3% in the subsequent 12 months to organizations that offer a plan in a payment area without an M+C plan since 1997, or in an area where all organizations announced withdrawal as of January 1, 2000. The BBRA reduced the exclusion period from five years to two years for organizations seeking to reenter the M+C Program after withdrawing. It allowed organizations to vary premiums, benefits, and cost sharing across individuals enrolled in the plan so long as these are uniform within segments comprising one or more M+C payment areas. BBRA provided for submission of adjusted community rates by July 1 instead of May 1. It provided that the aggregate amount of user fees collected would be based on the number of M+C beneficiaries in plans compared to the total number of beneficiaries. It also delayed implementation of the Medicare+Choice Competitive Bidding Demonstration Project, until 2002 at the earliest.

Medicare, Medicaid, and SCHIP Benefits Improvements, and Protection Act of 2000 (BIPA, P.L. 106-554)

BIPA established multiple floor rates, based on population and location. It applied a 3% minimum update in 2001, which returned to the existing law minimum update of 2% thereafter. BIPA increased the M+C payment rates for enrollees with ESRD to reflect the demonstration rate of social health maintenance organizations' ESRD capitation demonstrations. BIPA extended the current risk adjustment methodology until 2003 and, starting in 2004, began to phase-in a new risk adjustment methodology based on data from inpatient hospitals and ambulatory settings. It permitted M+C plans to offer reduced Medicare Part B premiums to their enrollees as part of providing any required additional benefits or reduced cost-sharing. It extended the application of the new entry bonus for M+C plans to include areas for which notification had been provided, as of October 3, 2000, that no plans would be available January 1, 2001. It required payment adjustments to M+C plans if a legislative change resulted in significant increased costs. It precluded the Secretary from implementing, other than at the beginning of a calendar year, regulations that imposed new, significant regulatory requirements on M+C organizations. BIPA required the Secretary to make decisions, within 10 days, approving or modifying marketing material used by M+C organizations, provided that the organization used model language specified by the Secretary. A provision allowed an M+C organization offering a plan in an area with more than one local coverage policy to use the local coverage policy for the part of the area that was most beneficial to M+C enrollees (as identified by the Secretary) for all M+C enrollees enrolled in the plan. BIPA expanded the M+C quality assurance programs for M+C plans to include a separate focus on racial and ethnic minorities. The Secretary was given authority to waive or modify requirements that hindered the design of, offering of, or enrollment in certain M+C plans, such as M+C plans under contract between M+C organizations and employers, labor organizations, or trustees of a fund established by employers and/or labor organizations. BIPA extended the period for Medigap enrollment for certain M+C enrollees affected by termination of coverage. It allowed individuals who enrolled in an M+C plan after the 10th day of the month to receive coverage beginning on the first day of the next calendar month. It permitted ESRD beneficiaries to enroll in another M+C plan if they lost coverage when their plan terminated its contract or reduced its service area. It required an M+C plan to cover post-hospitalization skilled nursing care through an enrollee's "home skilled nursing facility" in certain situations. BIPA mandated review of ACR submissions by the HCFA (now CMS) Chief Actuary.

Public Health Security and Bioterrorism Preparedness and Response Act (P.L. 107-188)

P.L. 107-188 moved CMS's annual announcement of M+C payment rates from no later than March 1 to no later than the second Monday in May, effective only in 2003 and 2004. It temporarily moved the deadline for plans to submit information about ACRs, M+C premiums, cost sharing, and additional benefits (if any) from no later than July 1 to no later than the second Monday in September in

2002, 2003, and 2004. It changed the annual coordinated election period from the month of November to November 15 through December 31 in 2002, 2003, and 2004. It allowed Medicare beneficiaries to make and change elections to an M+C plan on an ongoing basis through 2004. Then beginning in 2005, individuals would be able to make changes only on the more limited basis, originally scheduled to be phased in beginning in 2002.

Medicare Prescription Drug, Improvement, and Modernization Act of 2003 (MMA, P.L. 108-173)

In 2003, Congress passed the MMA, which made significant changes to Medicare's private plan option. For 2004, the MMA modified payment rates to plans. First, a fourth payment mechanism was added so that plans were paid the highest of the floor, minimum percentage increase, the blend or a new amount equal to 100% per capita fee-for-service for a beneficiary in original Medicare (including the value of indirect medical education.) Second, the blend payment type was not subject a budget neutrality provision. Third, beginning in 2004, the minimum percentage increase is the greater of either 2% or the growth in overall Medicare for the previous year. Beginning in 2005, the floor and blend payment types are eliminated; only the minimum percent increase amount, and in certain years, 100% of per capita FFS would be used to update payments.

Beginning in 2006, the MMA established a new payment methodology to pay private plans. Under the new payment system, Medicare continues to pay plans a fixed monthly amount per enrollee, but these monthly payments are determined, at least in part, by competitive bidding. The Secretary determines MA payments by comparing plan's estimated cost of providing covered Part A and B benefits (the bid) to the maximum amount Medicare is willing to pay a plan to provide covered Part A and B benefits (the benchmark). The benchmark amounts are the former per capita payment rates, and a revised update methodology applies. For plans that bid below the benchmark, the payment equals the bid amount plus 75% of the difference between the bid and the benchmark. The amount above the plan's bid may be used to provide additional benefits, reduce cost sharing, or may be applied towards the monthly Part B premium, or prescription drug premium. The remaining 25% is retained by the government. For plans that bid above the benchmark, the payment is the benchmark and enrollees must pay an additional premium equal to the amount by which the bid exceeds the benchmark.

Also beginning in 2006, MA regional plans are allowed to participate in the program. MA regional plans are coordinated care plans that cover both in- and out-of-network required services. Unlike local MA plans, regional MA plans are required to serve at least one entire region established by the Secretary. (The Secretary established 26 regions made up of states or multiple states.) Each regional plan is required to offer a maximum limit on out-of-pocket expenses and a unified Part A and B deductible. Payments for regional plans are also based on a competitive system described above, but for the regional program, the benchmark for each region is calculated using a statutory formula that includes a weighted average of plan bids for the region. The MMA established several incentives for private plans to participate in the regional program. Initially, 10 billion was provided in a stabilization fund, and additional amounts were to be added to the fund when regional plans bid below the benchmark. (Half of the 25% retained by the government when a regional plan bids below the benchmark is transferred to the MA regional plan stabilization fund.) During 2006 and 2007, Medicare was to share risk with MA regional plans if plan costs fall above or below a statutorily-specified risk corridor. Beginning in 2006, the Secretary was allowed to provide for an increased payment for certain hospitals that that contract with MA regional plans.

Beginning in 2006, beneficiaries can enroll in a Medicare Part D prescription drug plan whether they were in fee-for-service Medicare or enrolled in Medicare managed care. MA enrollees (except those in PFFS and MSAs) are required to get Part D benefits through their MA plan, if they want the Part D benefit.

MMA established the Medicare Special Needs Plan (SNP) option, which was intended to improve care coordination and service delivery for certain groups of Medicare beneficiaries. Under the SNP option, Medicare managed care plans are allowed to limit enrollment to certain types of beneficiaries such as dual eligibles. SNP plans may choose to better coordinate the care of dual eligibles by contracting with the state Medicaid agency to also provide Medicaid services, but SNP plans are not required to do so.

Starting in 2010, the MMA requires the Secretary to establish a program for the application of comparative cost adjustment (CCA) in CCA areas. The six-year program will begin January 1, 2010, and end December 31, 2015. The program is designed to test direct competition among local MA plans, as well as competition between local MA plans and original Medicare. The program will only occur in a limited number of statutorily qualifying areas.

Deficit Reduction Act (DRA, P.L. 109-171)

Starting in 2007, the DRA changed the way MA benchmarks are calculated to (1) exclude national adjustments for coding intensity, (2) exclude the budget neutral implementation of risk adjustment, (3) omit any adjustments accounting for errors in previous years' projections of the national per capita MA growth percentage, and (4) increase rates based on the MA growth percentage, as under current law. In the report language to the BBRA, Congress urged the Secretary to implement a more clinically based risk adjustment methodology (to supplement the demographic factors) without reducing overall payments to plans. To keep payments from being reduced overall, the Secretary applied a budget neutrality adjustment to risk adjusted rates. However, Administration studies show a difference in the reported health status of MA enrollees compared to the reported health status of beneficiaries in original Medicare. The exclusion of the budget neutral implementation of risk adjustment is being phased-in over four years (2007-2010).

Tax Relief and Health Care Act of 2006 (TRHCA, P.L. 109-432)

TRHCA created a special continuous open enrollment period for beneficiaries in original Medicare to join certain MA plans during 2007 and 2008 outside of the normal enrollment periods. It delayed the initial availability of funds from the MA Regional Plan Stabilization Fund until January 1, 2012, and reduced the amount of funds available to $3.5 billion.

P.L. 110-48 (An Act to Provide for the Extension of Transitional Medical Assistance, and Other Provisions)

P.L. 110-48 eliminated the special continuous open enrollment period added by TRHCA. It reduced the MA Regional Plan Stabilization Fund, to about $3.4 billion, and restricted the amount that could be spent in 2012 to $1.6 billion.

Medicare, Medicaid, and SCHIP Extensions Act of 2007 (MMSEA, P.L. 110-173)

The MMSEA extended the authority of Specialized Medicare Advantage Plans for Special Needs Individuals (SNPs) to restrict enrollment to special needs beneficiaries (defined as eligible enrollees who are institutionalized, are entitled to Medicaid, or would benefit from enrollment in a SNP) until January 1, 2010. Beginning January 1, 2008, it restricts the Secretary from designating other MA plans as SNPs and imposes a moratorium on new SNP plans until January 1, 2010. It extends for one year (to January 1, 2009) the length of time cost-based plans can continue to operate in an area with either two local or two regional MA plans in the same area. MMSEA eliminated $1.6 billion from the MA Regional Plan Stabilization Fund for 2012. It provided additional funding for State Health Insurance Assistance Programs, Area Agencies on Aging, and Aging and Disabled Resource Centers to provide information and counseling, and assistance to Medicare eligible individuals related to obtaining adequate and appropriate health coverage.

Medicare Improvements for Patients and Providers Act of 2008 (MIPPA, P.L. 110-275)

MIPPA requires the value of indirect medical education (IME) to be phased out of all benchmarks starting in 2010. The amount phased-out each year will be based on a ratio of (1) a specified percentage (0.60% in the first year), relative to (2) the proportion of per capita costs in original Medicare in the county that IME costs represent. The effect of the ratio is to phase out a higher proportion of IME costs in areas where IME makes up a smaller percentage of per capita spending in original Medicare. After 2010, the numerator phase-out percentage will be increased by 0.60 percentage points each year. This provision will not apply to PACE plans (Programs of All-Inclusive Care for the Elderly).

Starting in 2011, PFFS plans sponsored by employers or unions are required to establish contracted networks of providers to meet access requirements. Non-employer-sponsored MA PFFS plans are required to establish contracted networks of providers in network areas defined as areas having at least two plans with networks (such as health maintenance organizations [HMOs]). In areas without at least two network-based plans, the non-employer PFFS plans retain the ability to establish access requirements through establishing payment rates that are not less than those under original Medicare.

Beginning in January 1, 2010, PFFS and Medical Savings Account (MSA) plans are required to have a quality improvement program similar to other MA plans. Starting in 2011, data collection, reporting, and analysis requirements for PFFS and MSA plans may not exceed the requirements for local PPO plans, which are limited to those data from providers in the plan's contracted network, but not from out-of-network providers. In 2010, the data requirements for PFFS and MSA plans are limited to administrative data, but must be collected from both in-network and out-of-network providers.

MIPPA extends the time current Special Needs Plans (SNPs) may restrict enrollment to special needs individuals and extends the moratorium on the Secretary's authority to designate new SNPs until January 1, 2011. Starting January 1, 2010, all new enrollees in a SNP will be required to meet the definition of a special needs individual. For institutional SNPs, individuals living in the community who may need an institutional level of care are not eligible to enroll in the SNP unless it is determined by an entity other than the SNP using a state assessment tool that the individual needs an institutional level of care. Medicaid SNPs are required to have a contract with the state to provide Medicaid benefits, or arrange for benefits to be provided; Medicaid SNPs that do not comply with the contracting requirement will be permitted to participate in 2010, but will not be allowed to expand their service area. Further, Medicaid SNPs are required to provide prospective enrollees with descriptions of benefits and cost sharing under the Medicaid program and which are to be covered by the SNP. Chronic Care SNPs are required to comply with a revised definition of a Chronic Care SNP; the Secretary is also required to convene a panel of clinical advisors to determine which conditions meet the definition of a severe and disabling chronic condition. MIPPA requires all SNPs to comply with certain care management requirements, such as having an appropriate network of providers, performing enrollee health assessments, and arranging for interdisciplinary teams to manage care for enrollees. By no later than January 1, 2010, SNPs are required to collect and report data related to the care management requirements; the Secretary is required to conduct a review of SNPs in conjunction with its periodic financial audit of MA plans. Effective January 1, 2010, Medicaid Special Needs Plans (SNPs) serving dual eligible beneficiaries are prohibited from charging cost-sharing in excess of what would be permitted under Medicaid.

The MA Regional Plan Stabilization Fund is reduced to $1.00. A portion of the savings from the regional plan bidding process continues to flow into the Fund and is available for expenditures in 2014. MIPPA extends for one year—from

January 1, 2009, to January 1, 2010—the length of time reasonable cost plans may continue operating regardless of any other MA plans serving the area. It specifies that to prohibit the cost plan from participating after January 1, 2010, the two plans in the service area must be offered by different organizations. Finally, MIPPA modifies the minimum enrollment requirements for local or regional plans operating within the cost plan's service area. GAO is required to submit a report to Congress on the reasons why cost-based plans may be unable to become MA plans. MIPPA establishes new prohibitions on the marketing activities of MA plans and PDPs and their agents, brokers, or any third-party representatives. Except in instances when the beneficiary initiates contact, plans will be prohibited from soliciting beneficiaries door-to-door or on the phone. Cross-selling of non-health-related products, providing meals to prospective enrollees, marketing in areas where health care is delivered (i.e., physician offices or pharmacies), and using sales agents that are not state licensed are also prohibited. The provision requires that by November 15, 2008, the Secretary establish limitations on other plan marketing activities such as co-branding, marketing appointments with prospective enrollees, and agent compensation.

American Recovery and Reinvestment Act of 2009 (ARRA, P.L.111-5)

ARRA established bonus payments for selected Medicare Advantage HMO-affiliated eligible professionals and hospitals that were meaningful users of electronic health records.

End Notes

[1] http://www.medpac.gov/transcripts

[2] Medicare Payment Advisory Commission (MEDPAC), *Report to Congress: Medicare Payment Policy*, Chapter 3, Medicare Advantage, March 2008, p. 247, http://www.medpac.gov/chapters/Mar08_Ch03.pdf.

[3] Private fee for service plans (PFFS) are one type of private plan that may participate in the Medicare Advantage program. PFFS plans are defined as those that (1) reimburse providers on a fee-for-service basis without placing providers at a financial risk, (2) do not vary rates for a provider based on utilization related to that provider, and (3) do not restrict the selection of providers among those who are lawfully authorized to provide services and agree to the plan's terms and conditions of participation.

[4] Medicare Payment Advisory Commission (MEDPAC), *Report to Congress: Medicare Payment Policy*, Chapter 3, Medicare Advantage, March 2008, p. 247, http://www.medpac.gov/chapters /Mar08_Ch03.pdf.

[5] For the House Budget Committee, CMS Administrator Mark McClellan testified that MA plans brought "greater value to our overall health care system, in terms of enabling beneficiaries to get more up-to-date, higher-quality care at a lower cost." However, his argument defined costs more broadly than program by including beneficiary out-of-pocket costs as well. http://budget.house.gov/hearings/2007/06.28mcclellan_testimony

[6] Medicare Payment Advisory Commission, *Report to Congress*, March 2008, pp. 249-251, http://www.medpac.gov/chapters/Mar08_Ch03.pdf.

[7] Medicare Payment Advisory Commission, *Report to Congress*, March 2008, pp. 249-251, http://www.medpac.gov/chapters/Mar08_Ch03.pdf.

[8] CRS Report RL34592, *P.L. 110-275: The Medicare Improvements for Patients and Providers Act of 2008*

[9] Congressional Budget Office, *Budget Options*, December 2008, pp. 119-123, http://www.cbo.gov/ftpdocs/99xx/doc9925/12-18-HealthOptions.pdf.

[10] Robert A. Berenson, "From Politics to Policy: A New Payment Approach to Medicare Advantage," March 2008, pp. w156-w163.

[11] Congressional Budget Office, *Budget Options*, December 2008, pp. 119-123, http://www.cbo.gov/ftpdocs/99xx/doc9925/12-18-HealthOptions.pdf.

[12] Government Accountability Office, *Medicare Advantage Organizations: Actual Expenses and Profits Compared to Projections for 2005*, GAO-08-827R, June 24, 2008, http://www.gao.gov/new.items/d08827r.pdf, and Government Accountability Office, *Medicare Advantage organizations: Actual Expenses and Profits Compared to Projections for 2006*, GAO-09-132, December 8, 2008, http://www.gao.gov/new.items/d09132r.pdf.

[13] For a discussion on the interpretation of medical loss rations, please see, James C. Robinson, "Use and Abuse of the Medical Loss Ratio to Measure Health Plan Performance: This accounting tool was never intended to measure quality or efficiency," Health Affairs, July/August 1997, pp. 176-187.

[14] For a brief discussion of the Medicare Competitive Pricing Demonstrations during the 1990s, see, Robert A Berenson, "From Politics to Policy: A New Payment Approach to Medicare Advantage," *Health Affairs*, March 2008, pp. w160-w161.

In: Medicare Advantage: The Alternate Medicare … ISBN: 978-1-60876-031-2
Editors: Charles V. Baylis, pp.49-86

Chapter 2

MEDICARE ADVANTAGE: CHARACTERISTICS, FINANCIAL RISKS, AND DISENROLLMENT RATES OF BENEFICIARIES IN PRIVATE FEE-FOR-SERVICE PLANS

United States Government Accountability Office

WHY GAO DID THIS STUDY

Medicare Advantage (MA) plans are an alternative to the original Medicare fee-for-service (FFS) program. Private fee-for-service (PFFS) plans—one type of MA plan—give beneficiaries an option that is more like Medicare FFS than other MA plans, with a wider choice of providers and less plan management of services and providers. PFFS enrollment increased from about 35,000 beneficiaries in June 2004 to about 2.3 million in June 2008. This report compares PFFS plans to other MA plans and Medicare FFS in three areas: (1) characteristics of beneficiaries, (2) financial risks for beneficiaries who do not contact their plans before receiving services, and (3) disenrollment rates. To do this work, GAO reviewed materials from a selected sample of nine PFFS plan sponsors, analyzed Medicare data, and interviewed officials from CMS, which administers the Medicare program, and other organizations.

WHAT GAO RECOMMENDS

GAO recommends that CMS (1) investigate the extent to which PFFS beneficiaries face unexpected costs for not contacting their plan before receiving care, (2) ensure that CMS guidance on prior authorization reflects CMS policy, and (3) mail MA plan disenrollment rates to beneficiaries, as required by statute, and update rates on Medicare's Web site. CMS outlined the steps it was taking to respond to all three recommendations, but did not address how it would distribute disenrollment rates.

WHAT GAO FOUND

In April 2007, beneficiaries in PFFS plans tended to be healthier and generally younger than beneficiaries in other MA plans and Medicare FFS. Specifically, projected health care expenditures for PFFS beneficiaries were 7 percent less than the projected average for beneficiaries in other MA plans and 10 percent less than the projected average for beneficiaries in Medicare FFS. Beneficiaries in PFFS plans also generally were more likely than beneficiaries in other MA plans and Medicare FFS to reside in rural areas where fewer other MA plans were available. In addition, about 81 percent of beneficiaries who were new enrollees in PFFS plans were in Medicare FFS before enrolling in their plan, compared to 65 percent in other MA plans.

PFFS beneficiaries may have faced certain financial risks if they did not contact their plan before receiving services. These risks were generally not assumed by beneficiaries in other MA plans and Medicare FFS. Specifically, if beneficiaries or their providers did not contact their PFFS plans before obtaining a service to make sure it would be covered, beneficiaries unexpectedly may have had to pay for the entire cost of the service if coverage was later denied by their plan. CMS officials told GAO they did not have data on the extent to which PFFS beneficiaries were faced with such costs. Furthermore, some beneficiaries likely experienced higher out-of-pocket costs for covered services if they did not contact their plan before obtaining the services. For example, one sponsor of PFFS plans increased the share of the cost for which beneficiaries were responsible from 30 percent to 70 percent if the beneficiaries did not contact the plan before obtaining certain durable equipment. GAO found that some PFFS plans were inappropriately using the term prior authorization, which can involve denying service coverage if prior plan approval is not obtained, in their informational materials. CMS officials stated that PFFS plans should not have used this term because these plans were not permitted to deny service coverage due to lack of prior plan approval. However, CMS guidance on this issue has been inconsistent and sometimes incorrect.

From January through April 2007, beneficiaries in PFFS plans disenrolled at an average rate of 21 percent compared to 9 percent for other MA plans, and GAO concludes that CMS has not complied with statutory requirements to mail disenrollment rates to Medicare beneficiaries. Disenrollment rates can reflect factors such as beneficiary satisfaction and CMS is required by law to mail this information to Medicare beneficiaries to help them compare available MA plans in their area. Although CMS has not mailed disenrollment rates to beneficiaries since 2000, the agency did provide disenrollment rates through Medicare's Web site. However, this information was based on disenrollment in 2004 and 2005 and, given the enrollment growth since then, may not accurately reflect plans available to beneficiaries in 2008.

ABBREVIATIONS

AHIP	America's Health Insurance Plans
CBO	Congressional Budget Office
CMS	Centers for Medicare & Medicaid Services
CRS	Congressional Research Service
FFS	fee-for-service
HHS	Department of Health and Human Services
HMO	Health Maintenance Organization
MA	Medicare Advantage
MedPAC	Medicare Payment Advisory Commission
MIIR	Management Information Integrated Repository
MIPPA	Medicare Improvements for Patients and Providers Act of 2008
MOC	Medicare Options Compare
PBP	Plan Benefit Package
PFFS	private fee-for-service
PPO	Preferred Provider Organization
PSO	Provider-Sponsored Organization
SNP	Special Needs Plan

December 15, 2008
Congressional Requesters

Medicare Advantage (MA) plans are an alternative to original Medicare fee-for-service (FFS) in which private plans provide Medicare benefits to enrolled beneficiaries.[1] Enrollment in MA plans has grown substantially in recent years from about 4.7 million beneficiaries in June 2004 to 9.6 million—about 1 out of every 5 Medicare beneficiaries—as of June 2008. This increase in enrollment followed the enactment of the Medicare Prescription Drug, Improvement, and Modernization Act of 2003,[2] which among other things, resulted in increased payments to MA plans. MA plans are able to use the increased payments to offer more benefits and reduce beneficiary cost sharing relative to Medicare FFS. In addition, the increased payments allowed MA plans to expand into geographic areas where previously plan options had been very limited, resulting in more plan choices for beneficiaries.

Nearly half of the recent growth in MA enrollment, about 45 percent, occurred in one type of plan—private fee-for-service (PFFS) plans.[3] Enrollment in these plans increased from about 35,000 beneficiaries in June 2004 to about 2.3 million beneficiaries in June 2008. About one-quarter of beneficiaries enrolled in MA plans in June 2008 were enrolled in a PFFS plan, and 99 percent of Medicare beneficiaries in 2008 had access to a PFFS plan—up from 41 percent in 2005. The Congressional Budget Office (CBO) projects continued growth in PFFS and other MA plans through 2013, though at a slower pace.[4]

The growth in enrollment and availability of MA plans has financial implications for the Medicare program because the program pays more for beneficiaries in these plans than it would if they were in Medicare FFS. The federal government is projected to spend about $91 billion on the MA program in 2008.[5] According to the Medicare Payment Advisory Commission (MedPAC), in 2008, Medicare is projected to pay about 13 percent more for beneficiaries in MA plans overall and 17 percent more for beneficiaries in PFFS plans than what the program would have paid for these beneficiaries under Medicare FFS.[6]

PFFS plans are designed to offer beneficiaries an MA option that is more like Medicare FFS. Compared to other MA plans, PFFS plans generally offer a wider choice of providers and impose less plan management of health care services and providers. Unlike other types of MA plans, such as Health Maintenance Organizations (HMO) and Preferred Provider Organizations (PPO),[7] PFFS plans are not required to have networks of contracted providers if they pay providers Medicare FFS rates or higher.[8] Further, providers can agree to accept a PFFS beneficiary on a service-by-service basis. Almost all PFFS plans operate without networks.[9] Paying providers at Medicare FFS rates or higher suggests that beneficiaries in PFFS plans will have access to those providers who accept beneficiaries from Medicare's FFS program. However, there have been reports that, in some areas, it may be more difficult for beneficiaries to obtain care while in PFFS plans than it would be if they were in Medicare FFS.[10]

Under federal law, PFFS plans may not place providers at financial risk or restrict beneficiary access to providers.[11] The Centers for Medicare & Medicaid Services (CMS), the agency that administers the Medicare program,[12] prohibits PFFS plans—but not other types of MA plans—from requiring that providers or beneficiaries obtain plan approval before a service is furnished as a condition of coverage, a process known as prior authorization. However, sponsors of PFFS plans, like sponsors of other MA plans, must provide an advance coverage determination, should beneficiaries or their providers request one.[13] An advance coverage determination informs beneficiaries before they receive services whether the services will be covered and the amount that the beneficiary must pay with respect to such services. In finalizing regulations in 1998 for the MA program (then called the Medicare+Choice program), CMS considered requiring PFFS plan sponsors to mandate that providers who serve PFFS plan beneficiaries assume the responsibility for acquiring advance coverage determinations or risk being unable to charge beneficiaries if the plan later denied payments for the services.[14] CMS, however, determined that this beneficiary protection would be inconsistent with federal statutory provisions that prohibit PFFS plans from placing their providers at financial risk.

The rapid growth in PFFS plan enrollment highlights the need for more information about who is enrolling in, and disenrolling from, these plans. Specifically, if healthier beneficiaries are enrolling and staying in PFFS plans, this could leave other MA plans or the Medicare FFS program with sicker and potentially more costly beneficiaries. Also, if PFFS plans have high disenrollment rates compared to other MA plans, this could be an indicator of beneficiary dissatisfaction with access or quality of care or could indicate that other plans with more attractive benefit packages are available. In order to help Medicare beneficiaries compare and select MA plans, CMS is required by law to mail certain information to beneficiaries annually, including MA plan disenrollment rates for the previous 2 years to the extent that these disenrollment rates are available.[15]

Certain features of PFFS plans will change as a result of the Medicare Improvements for Patients and Providers Act of 2008 (MIPPA).[16] Beginning in 2011, PFFS plans will be required to form contracted networks of providers in areas that have at least two available network-based plans (such as HMOs or

PPOs).[17] In areas with fewer than two network-based plans, most PFFS plans will continue to have the option of operating without networks if they pay providers at Medicare FFS rates or higher.[18] In addition, beginning in 2010, PFFS plan sponsors will be required to have quality improvement programs for each plan and report related quality information to CMS.[19]

Given the uniqueness of PFFS plans and their rapid enrollment growth, you asked us to examine the characteristics of beneficiaries in these plans, PFFS plan features, and beneficiary disenrollment patterns. Our report addresses the following objectives: (1) compare the characteristics of beneficiaries in PFFS plans to the characteristics of beneficiaries in other MA plans and Medicare FFS; (2) describe the financial risks that beneficiaries in PFFS plans face, compared to beneficiaries in other MA plans and Medicare FFS, if they do not contact their plan prior to receiving services; and (3) compare the rates at which beneficiaries in PFFS plans disenroll to the rates for other MA plans and evaluate whether CMS met statutory requirements to mail disenrollment rates to beneficiaries.

To compare the characteristics of beneficiaries in PFFS plans, specifically age, gender, and residential location, to the characteristics of beneficiaries in other MA plans and Medicare FFS, we analyzed Medicare enrollment data for April 2007. We restricted our analysis to five types of MA plans that accounted for more than 99 percent of the approximately 7.8 million beneficiaries in MA plans at that time—PFFS plans, HMOs, local PPOs, regional PPOs, and Provider-Sponsored Organizations (PSO). After excluding plans that restrict enrollment and certain beneficiaries from our analysis, we analyzed data as of April 2007 for about 5.8 million beneficiaries in 1,998 MA plans and about 31.7 million beneficiaries in Medicare FFS.[20] To compare the health status of PFFS and other Medicare beneficiaries, we obtained plan-level risk scores from CMS, which are based on projected health care expenditures of plan beneficiaries and provide an indicator of the health status of the plans' beneficiaries. We also examined the type of Medicare coverage that MA beneficiaries held previously. For this analysis, we identified beneficiaries who were new to an MA plan type in April 2007 and examined their Medicare coverage in December 2006. MA plans that beneficiaries selected for 2007 generally took effect from January through April 2007.

To describe the financial risks that beneficiaries in PFFS plans face, compared to beneficiaries in other MA plans and Medicare FFS, if they do not contact their plan prior to receiving services, we reviewed relevant laws, regulations, documentation from CMS, and materials from nine PFFS plan sponsors interviewed that accounted for about 81 percent of PFFS enrollment in July 2007.[21] We reviewed 2008 plan benefit information provided to beneficiaries as well as provider terms and conditions of payment for 30 PFFS plans, accounting for more than half of each sponsor's total enrollment in PFFS plans. We reviewed 2008 plan benefit information provided to beneficiaries for 33 HMO or PPO plans operated by the same nine plan sponsors, accounting for more than half of each sponsor's total enrollment in other MA plans. We also interviewed officials from CMS and the plan sponsors. Information gathered from our review of the benefit information provided to beneficiaries for PFFS and other MA plans may not be representative of, or generalizable to, other MA plans offered by these and other plan sponsors that were not in our sample.

To compare the rates at which beneficiaries in PFFS plans disenroll to the rates for other MA plans, we used Medicare enrollment data for beneficiaries in PFFS and other MA plans in December 2006 and April 2007 to identify beneficiaries whose disenrollment took effect from January through April 2007.[22] We calculated disenrollment rates for each MA contract, which covered one or more MA plans of the same plan type.[23] To compare the health status of disenrollees to beneficiaries overall in PFFS and other MA plans, we used risk scores for 2006 as a proxy for health status. To evaluate whether CMS met statutory requirements to mail disenrollment rates to beneficiaries, we interviewed CMS officials, analyzed relevant federal laws and regulations, and reviewed disenrollment information CMS provided to Medicare beneficiaries through, for example, Medicare Options Compare (MOC) on Medicare's Web site.[24] MOC is a source of information through which beneficiaries can compare the quality, benefits, and premiums of MA plans.

We conducted interviews with CMS officials on the reliability of the CMS data used in our analysis. We also reviewed data documentation and performed certain data checks to ensure the data were reasonable and consistent. We determined that the data were sufficiently reliable for our purposes. We conducted our work from July 2007 through October 2008 in accordance with generally accepted government auditing standards. Those standards require that we plan and perform the audit to obtain sufficient, appropriate evidence to provide a reasonable basis for our findings and conclusions based on our audit objectives. We believe that the evidence obtained provides a reasonable basis for our findings and conclusions based on our audit objectives. See appendix I for more details on our scope and methodology.

RESULTS IN BRIEF

Beneficiaries in PFFS plans in April 2007 tended to be healthier and generally younger than beneficiaries in other MA plans and Medicare FFS, and were more likely to reside in rural areas where fewer other MA plan options were available. Specifically, beneficiaries in PFFS plans had projected health care expenditures—an indicator of health status—that were 7 percent less than the average for beneficiaries in other MA plans and 10 percent less than the average for beneficiaries in Medicare FFS. Beneficiaries in PFFS plans were less likely to be age 85 or older, and were more likely to reside in rural areas where, on average, beneficiaries had access to about 12 different PFFS plans but only about 4 other MA plans. In addition, about 81 percent of new enrollees in PFFS plans had been enrolled in Medicare FFS before enrolling in their plan, compared to about 65 percent of new enrollees in other MA plans.

If beneficiaries in PFFS plans did not contact their plans before obtaining services, they may have faced certain financial risks. These risks were generally not assumed by beneficiaries in other MA plans and Medicare FFS. Specifically, if beneficiaries in PFFS plans or their providers did not request an advance coverage determination from their plan before obtaining a service to ensure the service would be covered, beneficiaries unexpectedly may have had to pay for the entire cost of the service if coverage was later denied. However, beneficiaries in other MA plans and Medicare FFS generally had certain protections from this financial risk. CMS officials told us that they thought it was rare for PFFS beneficiaries to face unexpected costs of denied claims, but the agency did not have data on the extent to which this occurred. In addition, even when plans covered certain services, some PFFS beneficiaries likely experienced higher cost sharing if they or their providers did not notify their plans before receiving these services—a process called prenotification. For example, the coinsurance rate for certain durable medical equipment for one PFFS plan changed from 30 percent to 70 percent if beneficiaries or their providers did not prenotify their plan. In contrast, the other MA plans we reviewed did not have prenotification requirements, and Medicare FFS also had no such requirements. Furthermore, some PFFS plans' inappropriate use of the term prior authorization in their informational materials to describe beneficiary responsibilities for contacting their plan before receiving services may have confused beneficiaries and providers. According to CMS officials, PFFS plans should not have used the term prior authorization because PFFS plans cannot deny service coverage for lack of prior approval. However, CMS has provided inconsistent and sometimes incorrect guidance related to prior authorization for PFFS plans.

From January through April 2007, beneficiaries in PFFS plans disenrolled at an average rate of 21 percent compared to 9 percent for other MA plans, and we conclude that CMS did not comply with statutory requirements to mail information on MA plan disenrollment rates to beneficiaries. Beneficiaries who disenrolled from PFFS plans, on average, were sicker compared to all beneficiaries in PFFS plans, with projected health care expenditures that were about 6 percent higher than the average for all beneficiaries in these plans. The same pattern existed for other MA plans, though the difference was less pronounced. MA disenrollment rates varied depending on beneficiaries' age and location. For example, older beneficiaries in PFFS plans, such as those who were age 85 and older, disenrolled at higher rates, but this was not the case for other MA plans. PFFS beneficiaries in urban areas disenrolled at higher rates than beneficiaries in rural areas, while in other MA plans, beneficiaries in urban areas disenrolled at slightly lower rates. MA plan disenrollment rates can reflect differences across plans because of factors such as beneficiary satisfaction with care and out-of-pocket costs. CMS is required by law to mail disenrollment rates for the previous 2 years, to the extent available, to Medicare beneficiaries at least 15 days prior to each year's annual coordinated election period. CMS officials informed us that they had not mailed disenrollment rates to all Medicare beneficiaries since the fall of 2000. As these disenrollment rates were available to CMS, we conclude that CMS has not complied with statutory requirements to mail Medicare beneficiaries disenrollment rates for MA plans in their areas. CMS provided information on disenrollment rates and reasons for disenrollment to beneficiaries through MOC as of August 2008, but this information was based on data for 2004 and 2005.

We recommend that the Acting Administrator of CMS (1) investigate the extent to which beneficiaries in PFFS plans are faced with unexpected out-of-pocket costs due to the denial of coverage when they did not obtain an advance coverage determination from their plan; (2) ensure that CMS guidance on prior authorization accurately reflects CMS policy and that PFFS plan materials conform to CMS requirements; and (3) mail to Medicare beneficiaries MA plan disenrollment rates for the previous 2 years for MA plans that are or will be available in their areas, as required by statute, and update disenrollment rates provided to Medicare beneficiaries through MOC.

In commenting on a draft of this report, CMS described the steps it would take to address each of our three recommendations. In response to our recommendation that CMS investigate the extent to which beneficiaries in PFFS plans are faced with out-of-pocket costs due to the denial of coverage from their plan, CMS noted that it is examining coverage denials and complaints. In response to our recommendation that CMS correct its guidance related to prior authorization, CMS described several steps it has taken and plans to take, including issuing new guidance. In response to our recommendation that the agency mail disenrollment rates to beneficiaries and update the rates on its Web site, the agency commented that it had recently awarded a contract to obtain disenrollment rates and other performance metrics by late 2009. However, the agency did not indicate how it would provide disenrollment rate information to beneficiaries. We also obtained comments from representatives of America's Health Insurance Plans (AHIP), a national association that represents private health plans, who raised certain points they thought the report should have emphasized and made several other observations.

BACKGROUND

Medicare is the federal government's health insurance program that covers more than 44 million people age 65 and older and certain individuals who are disabled or have end-stage renal disease. Most Medicare beneficiaries can choose to receive covered services through Medicare FFS or through an MA plan if one is offered where they live.[25] Beneficiaries in Medicare FFS and in MA plans, including PFFS plans, pay monthly premiums and are responsible for cost sharing, which can be in the form of coinsurance (a percentage payment for a given service that a beneficiary must pay), a copayment (a standard amount a beneficiary must pay for a medical service), or a deductible (the amount a beneficiary must pay before Medicare FFS or an MA plan begins to pay). MA plans operate under annual contracts between MA plan sponsors and CMS and provide Medicare benefits in exchange for a monthly payment from CMS for each beneficiary enrolled in the plan.[26]

Beneficiaries can disenroll from MA plans during the annual coordinated election period, from November 15 through December 31 of a given year by enrolling in another plan or in Medicare FFS. Changes made during the annual coordinated election period take effect on January 1 of the following year. Beneficiaries can also disenroll from MA plans once during the open enrollment period, from January 1 through March 31 of a given year.[27] Changes made during this time period take effect on the first day of the month following the plan's receipt of the beneficiary's request.

BENEFICIARIES IN PFFS PLANS WERE HEALTHIER AND YOUNGER THAN BENEFICIARIES IN OTHER MA PLANS AND MEDICARE FFS AND DIFFERED IN OTHER WAYS

Relative to beneficiaries in other MA plans and Medicare FFS in April 2007, beneficiaries in PFFS plans were healthier, generally younger, and more likely to live in rural areas with fewer MA options. Specifically, beneficiaries in PFFS plans had projected health care expenditures—an indicator of health status—that were lower, on average, than those of beneficiaries in other MA plans and Medicare FFS. Beneficiaries in PFFS plans had projected health care expenditures that were 7 percent less than those of beneficiaries in other MA plans and 10 percent less than beneficiaries in Medicare FFS.

Beneficiaries in PFFS plans were generally more likely to be younger and reside in rural areas than beneficiaries in other MA plans and Medicare FFS (see table 1). PFFS plans had a smaller percentage of beneficiaries age 85 or older compared to other MA plans and Medicare FFS. Approximately 14 percent of PFFS beneficiaries lived in rural areas compared to 1 percent of beneficiaries in other MA plans and 10 percent of beneficiaries in Medicare FFS. Medicare beneficiaries in rural areas, on average, had access to about 12 different PFFS plan options, but only about 4 other MA plan options. In contrast, Medicare beneficiaries in urban areas had access to an average of about 13 PFFS plan options and about 12 other MA plan options. As a result, beneficiaries in rural areas might have been more likely to enroll in a PFFS plan because there were fewer other MA options available in those areas.

New enrollees in PFFS plans as of April 2007 were more likely than new enrollees in other MA plans to have been in Medicare FFS prior to enrollment but less likely to have been new to Medicare altogether or previously in a different type of plan. About 81 percent of new enrollees in PFFS plans were in Medicare FFS prior to joining their plan, compared to 65 percent of new enrollees in other MA plans (see table 2). About 6 percent of new PFFS enrollees were new Medicare beneficiaries prior to joining their plan, compared to about 13 percent of new enrollees in other MA plans. About 13 percent of new enrollees in PFFS plans were in a different type of plan before enrolling in their current plan, compared to 23 percent of new enrollees in other MA plans.

Table 1. Beneficiary Age, Gender, and Residence by Type of Medicare Coverage, 2007

	PFFS (percentage)	Other MA plans[a] (percentage)	Medicare FFS (percentage)
Age			
Under 65	16	9	17
65-74	52	45	41
75-84	26	34	30
85+	6	11	12
Gender			
Male	45	42	44
Female	55	58	56
Residence			
Urban[b]	86	99	89
Rural[c]	14	1	10

Sources: GAO analysis of CMS data and the Health Resources and Services Administration's Area Resource File.

Notes: Percentages may not sum to 100 due to rounding. Results are based on Medicare enrollment data as of April 2007 for 431 PFFS plans in which 1,304,288 beneficiaries were enrolled and 1,567 other MA plans in which 4,535,881 beneficiaries were enrolled.

[a] Other MA plans include HMOs, local PPOs, regional PPOs, and PSOs.

[b] Urban areas are defined as those areas that are classified either as Metropolitan Statistical Areas or Micropolitan Statistical Areas. Metropolitan Statistical Areas have at least one urbanized area with a population of 50,000 or more, plus adjacent territory that has a high degree of social and economic integration with the core as measured by commuting ties. Micropolitan Statistical Areas have at least one urban cluster with a population of at least 10,000 but less than 50,000, plus adjacent territory that has a high degree of social and economic integration with the core as measured by commuting ties.

[c] Rural areas are defined as those areas that are neither Metropolitan Statistical nor Micropolitan Statistical Areas and are not unknown.

Table 2. Type of Medicare Coverage before Enrollment for New Enrollees in PFFS or Other MA Plans, April 2007

	New enrollees in PFFS plans		New enrollees in other MA plans[b]	
Medicare coverage Before enrollment	**Number**	**Percentage**	**Number**	**Percentage**
Medicare FFS	467,458	81	309,572	65
New to Medicare	34,645	6	61,909	13
Other[a]	78,103	13	108,135	23
Total	**580,206**		**479,616**	

Sources: GAO analysis of CMS data.

Notes: Percentages may not sum to 100 due to rounding. New enrollees in PFFS and other MA plans were defined as beneficiaries who were in a given MA plan type (i.e., PFFS, HMO, local PPO, regional PPO, PSO) in April 2007 but who were not in that same plan type in December 2006.

[a] Includes enrollment in any type of Medicare private plan in which a beneficiary was enrolled in December 2006 that was different than their type of plan in April 2007.

[b] Other MA plans include HMOs, local PPOs, regional PPOs, and PSOs.

PFFS Beneficiaries May Have Faced Certain Financial Risks Generally Not Assumed by Beneficiaries in Other MA Plans and Medicare FFS

In contrast to most beneficiaries in other MA plans and Medicare FFS, beneficiaries in PFFS plans may have faced certain financial risks if they or their providers did not contact their plan before receiving services. Specifically, if PFFS beneficiaries or their providers did not obtain advance coverage determinations, which specified whether services would be covered and how much beneficiaries would have to pay, beneficiaries unexpectedly may have been responsible for the entire cost of the service if coverage was later denied by their PFFS plans as not medically necessary.[28] In addition, even if PFFS plans covered the services as medically necessary, some PFFS beneficiaries may have experienced substantially higher cost sharing if they or their providers did not contact their plans before receiving certain services. PFFS plans sometimes used the term prior authorization inappropriately to describe beneficiary or provider responsibilities for contacting their plans. CMS officials stated that PFFS plans should not have used this term because PFFS plans are not permitted to deny coverage for services when prior plan approval was not obtained. However, CMS guidance for PFFS plans related to prior authorization has been inconsistent and sometimes incorrect.

PFFS Beneficiaries Who Did Not Contact Their Plans to Determine Service Coverage before Receiving Services May Have Faced Unexpected Costs

If PFFS beneficiaries or their providers did not contact their plan before receiving a service to obtain an advance coverage determination, beneficiaries may have been responsible for the entire cost of the service if coverage for it was later denied by the plan because it was not medically necessary. Beneficiaries may have learned, from the information they received from their PFFS plan, whether a particular type of service would be covered, subject to a determination of medical necessity.[29] However, from that information, the beneficiary would not know whether the plan would determine a service to be medically necessary in a specific instance. To ascertain before a specific service was received whether it would be covered, beneficiaries or their providers may request an advance coverage determination from the PFFS plan.[30] CMS officials told us that they thought it was rare for beneficiaries in PFFS plans to face unexpected costs of denied claims, but they did not have data on the extent to which this occurs.[31]

Beneficiaries in other MA plans, such as HMOs and PPOs, generally had certain protections from unexpected costs when receiving services from network providers.[32] Pursuant to CMS policy, when beneficiaries in other MA plans seek care from network providers and these providers are required to fulfill plan procedures to ensure coverage of services, such as obtaining a referral or prior authorization, beneficiaries are held harmless financially when providers fail to take these steps.[33] In this circumstance, if beneficiaries in other MA plans reasonably believe that services would be covered, they would only be liable for their plan's cost sharing for the services, even if their plan later denies coverage. In addition, when these beneficiaries are responsible for taking steps to ensure coverage of services they receive from network providers, providers are required to inform beneficiaries of their responsibilities before providing these services. If the providers fail to do so, beneficiaries are responsible only for their plans' cost sharing for the services even if their plans later deny coverage. Because virtually all PFFS plans did not have provider networks, they did not provide these beneficiary protections.

Beneficiaries in Medicare FFS also had protection from the unexpected costs of claims that were denied when services provided were subsequently determined to be not medically necessary. Specifically, beneficiaries in Medicare FFS generally are protected from incurring financial liability if they do not receive an advance beneficiary notice notifying them when Medicare is expected to deny coverage for a given service because it was not medically necessary.

Some PFFS plans—plans administered by four of the nine PFFS plan sponsors we reviewed—required their providers, under the terms and conditions of the plans, to inform beneficiaries if a specific service was likely to be denied by the plan. However, these terms and conditions did not specify the penalty, if any, for not complying with this requirement. The terms and conditions of the remaining five plan sponsors did not require that providers notify beneficiaries if a service was likely to be denied by the plan.

Even When Certain Services Were Covered, Some PFFS Beneficiaries Likely Experienced Higher Cost Sharing If They Did Not Contact Their Plans before Receiving Such Services

Beneficiaries in some PFFS plans were responsible for higher cost-sharing amounts if they (or their health care providers) did not contact their plans in advance (a process called prenotification) before obtaining certain covered services. Under CMS policy, PFFS plans can vary cost sharing depending on whether beneficiaries (or their providers) have notified the plan before receiving certain services. Four of the nine PFFS plan sponsors in our review offered plans that charged higher cost sharing if prenotification did not occur for certain services, such as inpatient hospital stays, durable medical equipment, inpatient mental health services, and skilled nursing services. The specific services subject to prenotification requirements and the amount of additional cost sharing varied by PFFS plan and could have been substantial (see table 3), as the following examples illustrate.

- Three PFFS plan sponsors offered plans that required prenotification for inpatient hospital stays. Plans offered by two of the three PPFS plan sponsors increased required cost sharing by $100 to $150 per inpatient hospital admission without prenotification, while plans offered by the third sponsor required an additional $50 per day up to a maximum of $500 per admission.

- Four PFFS plan sponsors offered plans that required prenotification for durable medical equipment, and doubled, or more than doubled, beneficiary coinsurance rates if prenotification did not occur. One plan increased the coinsurance rate for durable medical equipment and prosthetic devices from 30 percent to 70 percent for items that cost more than $750 if beneficiaries or their providers did not prenotify. In these plans, for example, cost sharing for beneficiaries who purchased a power wheelchair for approximately $4,000 could increase from about $1,200 if they notified their plan to about $2,800 if they did not.
- Three PFFS plan sponsors offered plans that required prenotification for inpatient mental health stays and increased cost sharing in amounts ranging from $100 per admission to $50 per day up to a maximum of $500 if prenotification did not occur.
- One PFFS plan sponsor offered plans that required prenotification for skilled nursing facility stays and increased cost sharing by $50 per day up to a maximum of $500 if prenotification did not occur.

In contrast to PFFS plans, the other MA plans we reviewed did not appear to have prenotification requirements for services received from network providers. CMS officials noted that prenotification was generally unnecessary in HMOs, which accounted for about 89 percent of beneficiaries in other MA plans in April 2007, because HMOs typically had a primary care physician who authorized care for the beneficiary.[34] CMS officials also confirmed that Medicare FFS does not have prenotification requirements.

Administrators from one of the four plan sponsors that required prenotification told us that they did so for inpatient hospital stays and other services in order to help them identify beneficiaries for case and disease management and for discharge planning.[35] Administrators from another plan sponsor stated that they decided to require prenotificiation for durable medical equipment because the benefit typically had a high likelihood of abuse. A representative from another plan sponsor said that when the plan was prenotified it determined whether the equipment was medically necessary and informed the beneficiary of the potential financial liability that would be associated with the use or purchase of the durable medical equipment. The same representative noted that durable medical equipment was often determined to be not medically necessary.

Table 3. Examples of Cost Sharing with and without Prenotification In PFFS Plans Offered by Four Different Sponsors, 2008

	Cost sharing with prenotification	Cost sharing without prenotification
Plan A		
Inpatient hospital care[a]	Days 1–5: $150 copayment per day Days 6+: $0 copayment per day	Additional $50 per day up to $500 in additional payments
Durable medical equipment and prosthetic devices	30 percent coinsurance	70 percent coinsurance for equipment or a device that costs more than $750
Inpatient mental health	$500 copayment per hospital admission	Additional $50 per day up to $500 in additional payments
Skilled nursing facility	Days 1–20: $0 copayment per day Days 21–100: $50 copayment per day	Additional $50 per day up to $500 in additional payments
Plan B		
Inpatient hospital care[a]	$195 copayment per hospital admission	Additional $150 per hospital admission
Durable medical equipment and prosthetic devices	20 percent coinsurance	50 percent coinsurance for purchases of equipment or a device over $750
Inpatient mental health	Days 1–5 : $95 copayment per day Days 6–90: $0 copayment per day	Additional $50 each day up to $250 in additional payments
Skilled nursing facility	Days 1–20: $0 copayment per day Days 21–100: $100 copayment per day	NA—Prenotification not required
Plan C		
Inpatient hospital care[a]	$200 copayment per hospital admission	Additional $100 per hospital admission
Durable medical equipment	20 percent coinsurance	40 percent coinsurance for equipment that costs over $500
Inpatient mental health	$200 copayment per hospital admission	Additional $100 per admission
Skilled nursing facility	Days 1–15: $0 copayment per day Days 16–100: $80 copayment per day	NA—Prenotification not required
Plan D		
Inpatient hospital care[a]	Days 1–5: $100 copayment per day Days 6+: $0 copayment per day	NA—Prenotification not required
Durable medical equipment and prosthetic devices	20 percent coinsurance	50 percent coinsurance for equipment or a device over $750
Inpatient mental health	Days 1–5: $100 copayment per day Days 6+: $0 copayment per day	NA—Prenotification not required
Skilled nursing facility	Days 1–10: $0 copayment per day Days 11–100: $30 copayment per day	NA—Prenotification not required

Sources: PFFS plan sponsors.

[a] Includes substance abuse and rehabilitation services.

Some PFFS plans we reviewed inappropriately used the term prior authorization rather than prenotification in the informational materials they distributed to beneficiaries, which may have caused confusion about beneficiaries' financial risks. CMS officials stated that PFFS plans should not have used the term prior authorization because PFFS plans are not permitted to deny service coverage due to lack of prior plan approval.

Inconsistent information that CMS provided to PFFS plans may have contributed to some PFFS plans' inappropriate use of the term prior authorization. One source of CMS guidance—a CMS manual—incorrectly stated that PFFS plans' terms and conditions were required to indicate "whether the provider must obtain advance authorization from the PFFS organization before furnishing a particular service."[36] CMS officials acknowledged when we interviewed them in April 2008 that this statement was incorrect and should be deleted from its manual; however, as of August 2008 it had not been deleted.

Another source of inconsistent guidance from CMS was the data system that the agency used to obtain benefits information from PFFS and other MA plans. CMS officials explained that, prior to our inquiries, they did not realize that the Plan Benefit Package (PBP) software, which PFFS plans used to specify their benefits, did not allow plans to enter their prenotification information, but did allow plans to specify whether they had prior authorization requirements. As a result, some PFFS plans' summaries of benefits incorrectly indicated that these plans had prior authorization requirements. CMS officials said that they would update the PBP software for contract year 2010 to ensure that PFFS plans would be unable to specify prior authorization requirements and would make available a screen where PFFS plans could enter their prenotification information for specific services.

Following our inquiries on prior authorization and prenotification, CMS issued guidance to all PFFS plan sponsors in May 2008 through an operational policy memorandum to clarify its policy in these areas.[37] This policy memorandum reiterated that PFFS plans could not require prior authorization from providers or beneficiaries as a condition of coverage. Regarding prenotification, the policy memorandum clarified that PFFS plans could not impose penalties, but that they were permitted to offer cost-sharing reductions for complying with voluntary prenotification protocols.

PFFS Plans Had Relatively High Beneficiary Disenrollment Rates and CMS Did Not Comply with Statutory Requirements to Mail Current Rates

From January through April 2007, beneficiaries in PFFS plans disenrolled at an average rate that was more than twice that of other MA plans, and we conclude that CMS did not comply with statutory requirements to mail disenrollment rates to Medicare beneficiaries for the previous 2 years for MA plans in their area. Furthermore, information CMS has provided to beneficiaries on MA plan disenrollment rates and reasons for disenrollment is outdated.

Beneficiaries Disenrolled from PFFS Plans at a Higher Rate Than from Other MA Plans

Beneficiaries in PFFS plans were more than twice as likely to disenroll as beneficiaries in other MA plans from January through April 2007. PFFS beneficiaries disenrolled at an average rate of about 21 percent, compared to about 9 percent for beneficiaries in other MA plans. Disenrollment rates varied by plan, which could reflect plan-level differences in factors such as beneficiary satisfaction with care, service, and out-of-pocket costs. The range of disenrollment rates for PFFS plans—about 4 percent to 59 percent—was similar to the range of rates for other MA plans—about 2 percent to 54 percent.[38] However, PFFS beneficiaries were more likely than other MA beneficiaries to be in a plan with high disenrollment rates. For example, about 19 percent of PFFS beneficiaries were in plans that experienced disenrollment rates of 30 percent or more. In contrast, only 3 percent of other MA beneficiaries were in plans that experienced such high disenrollment rates. Approximately 15 percent of PFFS beneficiaries, but about 65 percent of other MA beneficiaries, were in plans that had disenrollment rates below 10 percent. (See figure 1.)

On average, disenrollees from PFFS plans were generally sicker compared to the average for all beneficiaries in PFFS plans. This pattern was also evident in other MA plans, although the average health status difference between disenrollees and all beneficiaries in these plans was less pronounced. Beneficiaries' risk scores indicated that the projected health care expenditures, on average, of disenrollees from PFFS plans were estimated to be about 6 percent higher than the average for all PFFS beneficiaries.[39] Similarly, beneficiaries who disenrolled from other MA plans had projected health care expenditures that were, on average, estimated to be about 3 percent higher compared to average projected health care expenditures for all beneficiaries in other MA plans.[40]

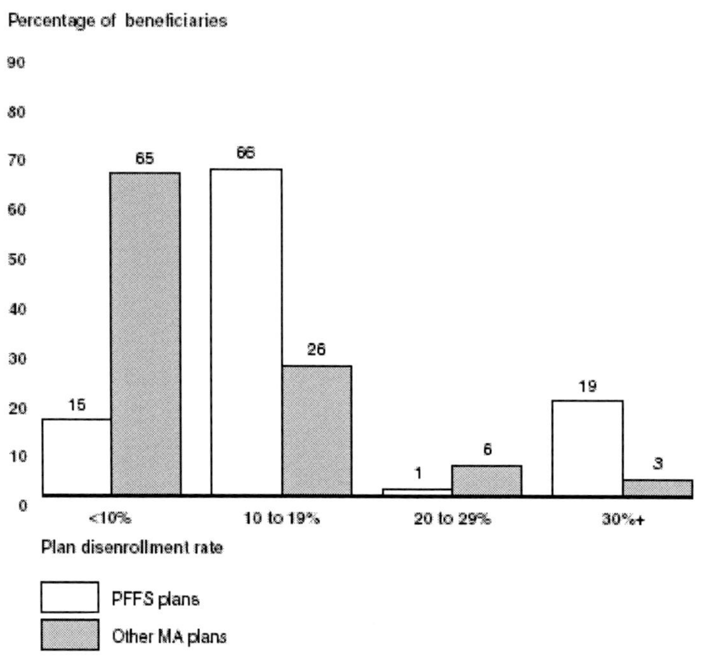

Source: GAO analysis of Medicare enrollment data for December 2006 and April 2007.

Notes: Percentages may not sum to 100 due to rounding. Results are based on disenrollment that occurred from January through April 2007 for 158 PFFS plans in which 805,734 beneficiaries were enrolled and 1,410 other MA plans in which 4,488,653 beneficiaries were enrolled in December 2006. The disenrollment rate for a given MA contract applies to all plans under that contract. Other MA plans include HMOs, local PPOs, regional PPOs, and PSOs.

Figure 1. Disenrollment Rates of PFFS and Other MA Plans for January through April 2007

PFFS disenrollment rates differed depending on beneficiaries' age group and location (see table 4). Older beneficiaries in PFFS plans tended to disenroll at higher rates. For example, PFFS beneficiaries age 85 and older had the highest disenrollment rate (about 25 percent) while beneficiaries younger than age 65 had the lowest disenrollment rate (about 18 percent). In contrast, there was no such relationship between age and disenrollment rates for other MA plans. Also, beneficiaries in PFFS plans who resided in urban areas were more likely than rural beneficiaries to disenroll, but this was not the case for other MA plans.

Table 4. Disenrollment Rates for PFFS and Other MA Plans by Beneficiary Characteristic, for January through April 2007

	PFFS plans	Other MA plans[a]
Beneficiaries overall	**21.3**	**8.9**
Age		
Under 65	18.2	9.8
65 to 74	20.3	9.1
75 to 84	24.1	8.3
85+	24.9	9.3
Residence		
Urban	22.0	8.9
Rural	17.2	10.6

Sources: GAO analysis of Medicare enrollment data for December 2006 and April 2007 and the Health Resources and Services Administration's Area Resource File.

Note: Results are based on disenrollment that occurred from January through April 2007 for 158 PFFS plans in which 805,734 beneficiaries were enrolled and 1,410 other MA plans in which 4,488,653 beneficiaries were enrolled in December 2006.

[a] Other MA plans include HMOs, local PPOs, regional PPOs, and PSOs.

CMS Did Not Comply with Statutory Requirements to Mail Current Disenrollment Rates to Medicare Beneficiaries

We conclude that CMS did not comply with statutory requirements to mail disenrollment rates to Medicare beneficiaries prior to the annual coordinated election period.[41] In creating the MA program (previously called the Medicare+Choice program), Congress required CMS to annually mail information to beneficiaries comparing MA plans, including PFFS plans.[42] The mailings were required to contain information about each MA plan available in a beneficiary's area, including beneficiary disenrollment rates for the previous 2 years, to the extent that these data were available.[43]

CMS officials informed us that they had not mailed disenrollment rate information to all Medicare beneficiaries since the Medicare & You 2001 handbook was sent in fall 2000, but more recent data were available. MA plan sponsors are required to provide CMS with disenrollment rates for beneficiaries who had been enrolled in their plans.[44] Although CMS did not respond to our questions about whether MA plan sponsors complied with requirements to provide CMS with disenrollment rates, CMS does have the information needed to calculate current disenrollment rates by using Medicare enrollment data. We used Medicare enrollment data from CMS to calculate disenrollment rates presented in this report for January through April 2007 and also in previous reports in 1996 and 1998.[45]

In response to our inquiries, CMS officials stated that there is no requirement to mail disenrollment rates to Medicare beneficiaries, but did not provide any explanation for the agency's position. We, however, disagree as under federal law, prior to each annual coordinated election period, CMS is required to provide to Medicare beneficiaries disenrollment rates for plans in their area to the extent these rates are available. Because we concluded that disenrollment rates for MA plans were available, CMS was required to include relevant disenrollment rates in annual mailings to Medicare beneficiaries to enable them to make informed choices about their Medicare coverage.

CMS published disenrollment rates and reasons for disenrollment through MOC on Medicare's Web site. As of August 2008, this information was available through MOC based on data for 2004 and 2005. However, given the recent growth in PFFS plans, from about 109,000 beneficiaries in June 2005 to about 2.3 million beneficiaries in June 2008, disenrollment rates and reasons for disenrollment based on disenrollment in 2004 and 2005 may not accurately represent the experience of PFFS plans available to beneficiaries in 2008. CMS officials stated that information on beneficiaries' reasons for disenrollment is necessary to understand the underlying differences in disenrollment rates across plans. Nonetheless, CMS officials said that the disenrollment reasons survey was discontinued after 2005 due to budget constraints. A CMS official also noted that providing disenrollment rates without reasons for disenrollment would be misleading because one would not know the extent to which beneficiaries left a plan, for example, because another plan was less expensive or due to poor quality care. We disagree with CMS's position. Although it would be useful to know the reasons behind beneficiaries' disenrollment decisions, disenrollment rates alone can provide useful relative information about MA plans and prompt beneficiaries to investigate plans further.

Conclusions

The substantial enrollment growth in PFFS plans shows that these plans are an attractive option for Medicare beneficiaries. Yet, beneficiaries in these plans may have faced unexpected out-of-pocket costs if plans denied coverage for services for which beneficiaries or their providers had not obtained an advance coverage determination. While officials from CMS did not believe that PFFS plans often denied services unexpectedly for not being medically necessary, it is important to determine the extent to which such denials occur. Having this knowledge would inform CMS and policy makers about whether additional protective measures or beneficiary educational efforts are warranted. It is also important that beneficiaries have accurate and current information about MA plans' policies and procedures. As such, ensuring that prior authorization guidance is accurate will help beneficiaries and providers better understand the obligations and financial risks associated with PFFS plans. Similarly, providing beneficiaries with current information about MA plan disenrollment rates would help them make more informed choices when considering enrolling in an MA plan.

Recommendations for Executive Action

We recommend that the Acting Administrator of CMS take the following three actions:

- investigate the extent to which beneficiaries in PFFS plans are faced with unexpected out-of-pocket costs due to the denial of coverage when they did not obtain an advance coverage determination from their plan;
- ensure that CMS guidance on prior authorization accurately reflects CMS policy and that PFFS plan materials conform to CMS requirements; and
- mail to Medicare beneficiaries MA plan disenrollment rates for the previous 2 years for MA plans that are or will be available in their areas, as required by statute, and update disenrollment rates provided to Medicare beneficiaries through MOC.

Agency and Other External Comments

We provided a draft of this report to CMS and AHIP for comment. CMS provided us with written comments that are reprinted in appendix II, and representatives from AHIP provided us with oral comments.

CMS Comments

CMS stated that beneficiaries may have more certainty that a particular service will be covered if that service is obtained from a provider in a plan's network. As a consequence, CMS stated that it is important for beneficiaries in non-network plans (such as virtually all PFFS plans) to understand their rights and obligations. CMS advised that beneficiaries in non-network plans may want to consider obtaining advance determinations from their plans in appropriate circumstances. CMS said that it would continue to work closely with Congress, GAO, beneficiary advocacy groups, and other interested parties to ensure that beneficiaries receive appropriate health care and do not incur unexpected financial risks.

CMS outlined the steps that it was taking, or planned to take, in response to each of our three recommendations. In response to our recommendation that CMS investigate the extent to which beneficiaries in PFFS plans are faced with out-of-pocket costs due to the denial of coverage when they did not obtain an advance coverage determination from their plan, CMS is examining coverage denials and complaints, and will be collecting new information from plans and refining its complaint tracking module to support this effort. In response to our recommendation that CMS ensure prior authorization guidance accurately reflects CMS policy, the agency described several steps it has already taken and planned to take to address the inaccuracies, including providing new guidance, modifying the PBP, and providing model terms and conditions that PFFS plans will be required to use in 2009. In response to our recommendation that CMS mail disenrollment rates to Medicare beneficiaries and update disenrollment rates through MOC, the agency commented that it had recently awarded a contract to obtain disenrollment rates and other performance metrics by late 2009. However, the agency was silent as to how it would distribute information on MA plan disenrollment rates to beneficiaries.

AHIP Comments

In general, AHIP representatives thought the report could better highlight certain points related to prenotification, MIPPA, and case management, and AHIP representatives made several observations about other aspects of the report.

AHIP representatives stated that, while our presentation of prenotification requirements was accurate, the report should have more clearly stated that we did not know the extent to which beneficiaries actually faced higher cost sharing as a result of not fulfilling prenotification requirements. They also stated that our discussion of MIPPA should have occurred earlier in the report given the potential impact of this legislation on PFFS plans, and suggested that our finding that all nine PFFS organizations in our study provided either case management or disease management services should have been given greater prominence in the report. We believe our methodology and findings regarding prenotification are clearly presented in the report and do not agree that clarifications are warranted. We also believe the placement and emphasis on MIPPA and case and disease management are appropriate given the focus and timing of our work.

AHIP representatives made several other observations they thought might help clarify aspects of the report. They explained that prenotification was originally intended to protect beneficiaries by providing them with an incentive to contact their plan to determine whether a service was covered before the service was rendered. AHIP representatives informed us that CMS had posted standard terms and conditions on its Web site that would help to address use of incorrect terms by the industry. They also stated that one explanation for our finding that beneficiaries in PFFS plans were younger on average could be that younger beneficiaries were more likely to try new types of plans. In addition, AHIP representatives emphasized the importance of collecting information about beneficiary reasons for disenrollment and endorsed making this information available to beneficiaries.

As agreed with your offices, unless you publicly announce the contents of this report earlier, we plan no further distribution until 30 days from the report date. At that time, we will send copies to the Acting CMS Administrator, appropriate congressional committees and others. The report also will be available at no charge on the GAO Web site at http://www.gao.gov/ .

If you or your staff have any questions about this report, please contact me at (202) 512-7114 or cosgrovej@gao.gov. Contact points for our Offices of Congressional Relations and Public Affairs may be found on the last page of this report. GAO staff who made major contributions to this report are listed in appendix III.

James C. Cosgrove
Director, Health Care

List of Requesters

The Honorable John D. Dingell
Chairman
Committee on Energy and
Commerce House of Representatives

The Honorable Henry A. Waxman
Chairman
Committee on Oversight and Government Reform
House of Representatives

The Honorable Charles B. Rangel
Chairman
Committee on Ways and Means
House of Representatives

The Honorable Frank J. Pallone, Jr.
Chairman
Subcommittee on Health
Committee on Energy and Commerce
House of Representatives

The Honorable Pete Stark
Chairman Subcommittee on Health
Committee on Ways and Means
House of Representatives

APPENDIX I: SCOPE AND METHODOLOGY

This appendix explains the scope and methodology that we used to address our reporting objectives that (1) compare the characteristics of beneficiaries in private fee-for-service (PFFS) plans to the characteristics of beneficiaries in other MA plans and Medicare FFS; (2) describe the financial risks that beneficiaries in PFFS plans face, compared to beneficiaries in other Medicare Advantage (MA) plans and Medicare fee-for-service (FFS), if they do not contact their plan prior to receiving services; and (3) compare the rates at which beneficiaries in PFFS plans disenroll to the rates for other MA plans and evaluate whether the Centers for Medicare & Medicaid Services (CMS) met statutory requirements to mail disenrollment rates to beneficiaries.

To compare the characteristics of beneficiaries in PFFS plans, specifically age, gender, and residential location, to the characteristics of beneficiaries in other MA plans and Medicare FFS, we used Medicare enrollment data from CMS for April 2007 from the Management Information Integrated Repository (MIIR) database and data from CMS on the average risk score for each MA plan in 2007, which provide an indicator of the health status of the plan's beneficiaries.[46] We focused our analysis on beneficiaries enrolled in five types of MA plans as of April 2007 that accounted for more than 99 percent of the approximately 7.8 million beneficiaries in MA plans at that time—PFFS plans and four other types of MA plans—Health Maintenance Organizations (HMO), Local Preferred Provider Organizations (PPO), regional PPOs, and Provider-Sponsored Organizations (PSO).[47] Among beneficiaries in the five MA plan types in our analysis, we excluded those (1) who were in plans that have enrollment restrictions (i.e., employer plans, Special Needs Plans (SNP), and plans that only cover Medicare Part B services) and (2) who live outside the 50 states, the District of Columbia, and Puerto Rico. After implementing these exclusions, we analyzed data as of April 2007 for 1,304,288 beneficiaries in 431 PFFS plans, 4,535,881 beneficiaries in 1,567 other MA plans, and 31,680,824 beneficiaries in Medicare FFS.[48] We used the Health Resources and Services Administration's Area Resource File for 2006 to obtain data on counties' level of urbanization.[49] We defined new enrollees in PFFS and other MA plans as beneficiaries who were in a given MA plan type in April 2007, based on data from the MIIR database, but who were not in that same plan type in December 2006. To compare the health status of beneficiaries in PFFS plans, other MA plans, and Medicare FFS, we used plan-level risk scores from CMS as a proxy for health status. After excluding beneficiaries in employer plans, SNPs, and plans that only cover certain Medicare FFS services as described above, we analyzed risk scores for 430 PFFS plans in which 1,371,169 beneficiaries were enrolled and 1,576 other MA plans in which 4,610,368 beneficiaries were enrolled as of July 2007.

To describe the financial risks that beneficiaries in PFFS plans face, compared to beneficiaries in other MA plans and Medicare FFS, if they do not contact their plan prior to receiving services, we reviewed relevant laws, regulations, documentation from CMS, and materials from nine PFFS plan sponsors interviewed that accounted for about 81 percent of PFFS enrollment in July 2007.[50] We reviewed plan benefit information for 2008 provided to beneficiaries as well as provider terms and conditions of payment for 30 PFFS plans, accounting for more than half of each sponsor's total PFFS plan enrollment. We reviewed plan benefit information for 2008 provided to beneficiaries for 33 HMO or PPO plans operated by the same nine plan sponsors, accounting for more than half of each sponsor's total enrollment in other MA plans. If the plan's benefit information provided to beneficiaries explicitly stated that beneficiaries would face higher cost sharing for certain services if they or their provider did not notify the plan before receiving such services, we considered that plan to have a prenotification requirement. We also interviewed officials from CMS and the plan sponsors. Information gathered from our review of the benefit information provided to beneficiaries for PFFS and other MA plans may not be representative of, or generalizeable to, other types of plans offered by these plan sponsors or to other PFFS and other MA plans that were not in our sample.

To compare the rates at which beneficiaries in PFFS plans disenroll to the rates for other MA plans, we used Medicare enrollment data from the MIIR database for 6,913,780 beneficiaries in MA plans in December 2006. Because MA plan selections for 2007 generally take effect from January through April 2007, we identified disenrollees as beneficiaries who were covered under a given MA contract in December 2006 but were no longer covered under that contract in April 2007 based on Medicare enrollment data.[51] Because we calculated disenrollment at the MA contract level, we did not address the extent to which beneficiaries transferred from one plan to another within an MA contract. We chose to calculate disenrollment rates at the MA contract level, rather than at the MA plan level, for two reasons: (1) transferring from one plan to another within a contract can occur for administrative reasons and therefore may not reflect beneficiary decisions, and (2) a beneficiary's decision to transfer, for example, from a zero premium plan to a plan within the same MA contract that charges a premium and has a richer benefit package does not suggest dissatisfaction with the type of MA plan or the sponsor that administers it. We calculated disenrollment rates for each MA contract as the total number of beneficiaries who disenrolled from their MA contract divided by total enrollment in that contract.[52] The disenrollment rate for an MA contract applies to all plans under that contract.

We did not include beneficiaries in disenrollment rate calculations if they disenrolled involuntarily due to factors such as death, loss of Medicare eligibility, moving out of their MA contract's service area, or to administrative factors such as a change in their MA contract's service area or a termination of their MA contract or plan.[53] After excluding beneficiaries (1) in certain plans and locations as described above and (2) in contracts or plans that were terminated in 2006 or 2007, we analyzed data for 158 PFFS plans accounting for 805,734 beneficiaries and 169,465 disenrollees and for 1,410 other MA plans accounting for 4,488,653 beneficiaries and 392,704 disenrollees.

We used risk scores for 2006—an indicator of projected health care expenditures—to compare the health status of disenrollees to beneficiaries overall in PFFS and other MA plans. To estimate average risk scores of disenrollees from PFFS and other MA plans, we used 2006 beneficiary-level risk scores for 169,271 beneficiaries who disenrolled from PFFS plans and for 391,126 beneficiaries who disenrolled from other MA plans from January through April 2007. To estimate the average risk scores of beneficiaries overall in these plans, we used 2006 plan-level risk scores, which are based on 725,110 beneficiaries in 154 PFFS plans and 4,421,308 beneficiaries in 1,400 other MA plans in July 2006, and weighted each plan's risk score by its July 2006 enrollment. According to a CMS official, MA plans' risk scores generally decline over the course of a year, so a plan's risk score based on beneficiaries in the plan in July 2006 could be higher than it would have been based on beneficiaries in the plan in December 2006.[54] As a result, the actual percentage difference between the average projected health care expenditures for disenrollees in PFFS and other MA plans and beneficiaries overall in these plans may be larger than our estimates indicate. To evaluate whether CMS met statutory requirements to mail disenrollment rates to beneficiaries, we interviewed CMS officials, analyzed relevant federal laws and regulations, and reviewed information CMS provided to Medicare beneficiaries through, for example, Medicare Options Compare (MOC) on Medicare's Web site.[55]

APPENDIX II: COMMENTS FROM THE CENTERS FOR MEDICARE & MEDICAID SERVICES

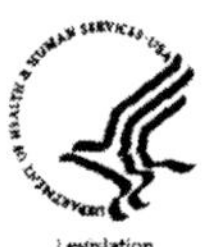

DEPARTMENT OF HEALTH & HUMAN SERVICES OFFICE OF THE SECRETARY

Assistant Secretary for Legislation

Washington, DC 20201

DEC 01 2008

James Cosgrove
Director, Health Care
U.S. Government Accountability Office
441 G Street N.W.
Washington, DC 20548

Dear Mr. Cosgrove:

Enclosed are comments on the U.S. Government Accountability Office's (GAO) report entitled: "Medicare Advantage: Characteristics, Financial Risks, and Disenrollment Rates of Beneficiaries in private Fee-for-Service Plans" (GAO 09-25).

The Department appreciates the opportunity to review this report before its publication.

Sincerely,

for Vincent J. Ventimiglia, Jr.
Assistant Secretary for Legislation

Attachment

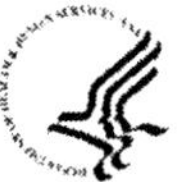

DEPARTMENT OF HEALTH & HUMAN SERVICES

Centers for Medicare & Medicaid Services

200 Independence Avenue SW
Washington, DC 20201

DATE: NOV 2 5 2008

TO: Vincent J. Ventimiglia, Jr.
Assistant Secretary for Legislation
Department of Health and Human Services

FROM: Kerry Weems
Acting Administrator

SUBJECT: Government Accountability Office (GAO) Draft Report: "Medicare Advantage: Characteristics, Financial Risks, and Disenrollment Rates of Beneficiaries in Private Fee-for-Service Plans" (GAO-09-25)

Thank you for the opportunity to review and comment on the GAO Draft Report titled "MEDICARE ADVANTAGE: Characteristics, Financial Risks, and Disenrollment Rates of Beneficiaries in Private Fee-for-Service Plans" (GAO-09-25). The Centers for Medicare & Medicaid Services (CMS) is committed to ensuring that Medicare beneficiaries receive appropriate health care services.

There are certain important elements that beneficiaries in a health plan offering coverage through non-network providers must consider. The report highlights one of those elements - that using network providers may provide a greater degree of certainty that all procedural claims rules will be followed and a particular service will in fact be covered by the plan. Thus, it is important for beneficiaries in non-network plans to understand their rights and obligations, and they may want to consider obtaining advance determinations from their plans in appropriate circumstances.

Consistent with GAO's recommendations, CMS is reviewing the adequacy of information that Medicare Advantage (MA) private fee-for-service (PFFS) plans have provided with respect to advance coverage determinations and notices. CMS has also clarified and is monitoring compliance with our rules that prohibit prior authorization for covered services.

The CMS will continue to work closely with Congress, GAO, beneficiary advocacy groups, and other interested parties to ensure that beneficiaries receive appropriate health care and do not incur unexpected financial risks.

Page 2 - Vincent J. Ventimiglia, Jr.

GAO Recommendation

The GAO recommends CMS investigate the extent to which beneficiaries in PFFS plans are faced with unexpected out-of-pocket costs due to the denial of coverage where they did not obtain an advance coverage determination from their plan.

CMS Response

We are looking at coverage denials and complaints to determine whether there may be a problem with the adequacy of communication between plans and members, and whether it suggests that beneficiaries are not sufficiently taking advantage of their rights to receive an advance coverage determination.

On October 3, 2008, CMS published a summary of proposed data collection requirements for Medicare Advantage organizations (MAOs) in the *Federal Register*. CMS proposed to collect organization determinations and reconsiderations data from PFFS plans as well as other MA plans to ensure that PFFS plans are not inappropriately denying plan-covered services. CMS will monitor the number of denial of coverage cases generated by PFFS plans on a quarterly basis, and will release the final data collection requirements in December 2008.

The CMS is also refining its process for prioritizing beneficiary complaints to ensure that access to care complaints entered into the complaint tracking module (CTM) receive first priority. We believe a systematic monitoring of complaints will enable CMS to identify those PFFS plans as well as other MA plans that are inappropriately denying their enrollees health care services.

In cases of denied coverage of plan-covered services, the beneficiary has recourse to a comprehensive and well established appeals process that furnishes enrollees access to an independent review entity and additionally an administrative law judge (see 42 CFR Subpart M). Also, the plan is obligated to provide the beneficiary with a Notice of Denial of Medical Coverage, which explains the beneficiary's appeal rights and why the service was denied coverage.

PFFS plans must cover all medically necessary services covered by Original Medicare, in addition to any supplemental services covered by the plan. PFFS plans must use Medicare's coverage rules to decide what services are medically necessary. If a service is medically necessary under Original Medicare, then the PFFS plan must cover the service. PFFS plans must ensure there is no difference in access to covered services between beneficiaries enrolled in a PFFS plan and beneficiaries enrolled in Original Medicare.

GAO Recommendation

The GAO recommends CMS ensure guidance regarding prior authorization accurately reflects CMS policy and that PFFS plan materials conform to CMS requirements.

Page 3 - Vincent J. Ventimiglia, Jr.

CMS Response

We concur with the GAO's recommendation and have already taken several steps to ensure that guidance to plans accurately reflects CMS' policy that PFFS Plans cannot require prior authorization as a condition of coverage and PFFS plan materials conform to CMS requirements.

- In the 2009 Call Letter released on March 17, 2008, CMS described its policy that PFFS plans may not require enrollees or providers to obtain prior authorization from the plan as a condition of coverage. CMS reiterated this policy in a memorandum to PFFS plans that was released on May 29, 2008.
- CMS modified the Plan Benefit Package (PBP) for contract year 2010 so that PFFS plans are no longer able to indicate that they have prior authorization requirements.
- On September 12, 2008, CMS released a memorandum to PFFS plans titled "Instructions For Model Private Fee-For-Service Terms And Conditions of Payment". This memorandum provided PFFS plans with a model terms and conditions of payment, which reiterated CMS' policy that prior authorization cannot be required as a condition of coverage when medically necessary, plan-covered services are furnished to enrollees. CMS also indicated in this memorandum that, effective January 1, 2009, it expects all PFFS plans to have implemented the model terms and conditions of payment.
- We are currently in the process of revising the Medicare Managed Care Manual to accurately reflect our policy on prior authorization for PFFS plans.
- CMS will also review plan materials to ensure plan materials accurately describe CMS' prior authorization requirements.

GAO Recommendation

The GAO recommends CMS comply with statutory requirements to mail to Medicare beneficiaries MA plan disenrollment rates for the previous two years for MA plans that are or will be available in their areas, and update disenrollment rates provided to Medicare beneficiaries through MOC.

CMS Response

The CMS has recently awarded a contract to develop performance metrics for Medicare Advantage plans, including PFFS plans. CMS will have information on PFFS disenrollment rates from this contract by late 2009.

Again, we thank you for the opportunity to review and comment on this draft report.

End Notes

[1] Medicare is the federally financed health insurance program for persons age 65 and older, certain individuals with disabilities, and individuals with end-stage renal disease. Medicare Part A covers hospital and other inpatient stays. Medicare Part B is optional insurance, and covers hospital outpatient, physician, and other services. Medicare Parts A and B are known as Medicare FFS.

[2] Medicare Prescription Drug, Improvement, and Modernization Act of 2003, Pub. L. No. 108-173, §§ 211, et seq., 117 Stat. 2066, 2176-2207 (2003) (codified, as amended, at 42 U.S.C. §§ 1395w-21, et seq.).

[3] PFFS plans were first authorized for Medicare beneficiaries under the Balanced Budget Act of 1997, Pub. L. No. 105-33, § 4001, 111 Stat. 251, 275-327 (1997) (codified, as amended, at 42 U.S.C. §§ 1395w-21, et seq.).

[4] CBO, *Cost Estimate, Medicare Improvements for Patients and Providers Act of 2008* (July 23, 2008).

[5] CBO, *The Medicare Advantage Program: Trends and Options*, Testimony of Peter R. Orszag before the Subcommittee on Health, Committee on Ways and Means, U.S. House of Representatives (Mar. 21, 2007).

[6] Medicare Payment Advisory Commission (MedPAC), *Report to the Congress: Medicare Payment Policy* (Washington, D.C.: March 2008).

[7] We use the term other MA plans to refer to network-based HMOs, PPOs, and Provider-Sponsored Organizations (PSO). Beneficiaries in HMOs are generally restricted to seeing providers within a network. Beneficiaries in regional and local PPOs can see both in-network and out-of-network providers but usually must pay higher cost-sharing amounts if they use out-of-network services. A regional PPO serves an entire state or multiple states, whereas local PPOs may serve a county, partial county, or multiple counties. PSOs are operated by a provider or a group of affiliated providers where a substantial proportion of health care services are provided directly through the provider or providers.

[8] A PFFS plan sponsor must demonstrate to the Secretary of Health and Human Services that it has a sufficient number and range of providers willing to furnish services under the plan by either (1) the plan establishing provider payment rates that are not less than the rates that apply under Medicare FFS, (2) the plan establishing contracts or agreements with a sufficient number and range of providers to furnish the services covered under the PFFS plan, or (3) a combination of the two options. 42 U.S.C. § 1395w-22(d)(4). Hereafter in this report, we refer to organizations offering MA plans, including PFFS plans, as plan sponsors.

[9] PFFS plans may treat providers as if they have a written contract with the plan if before rendering covered services, the provider has been informed of the beneficiary's enrollment in the plan and knows of, or had a reasonable opportunity to obtain, the terms and conditions of the plan. 42 U.S.C. § 1395w-22(j)(6).

[10] Congressional Research Service (CRS), *CRS Report for Congress: Private Fee for Service (PFFS) Plans - How They Differ From Other Medicare Advantage Plans* (Washington, D.C.: 2007).

[11] PFFS plans must pay providers at a rate determined by the plan on a fee-for-service basis without placing the provider at financial risk. The plans also may not vary the rates for a provider based on the utilization of that provider's services nor restrict enrollees' choices among providers who are lawfully authorized to provide services and agree to accept the plan's terms and conditions of payment. 42 U.S.C. § 1395w-28(b)(2).

[12] CMS is an agency within the Department of Health and Human Services (HHS), to which HHS has delegated the responsibility for administering the Medicare program.

[13] MA plan sponsors must have procedures for making timely determinations on whether a beneficiary is entitled to receive a service and the amount, if any, the beneficiary must pay for the service. 42 U.S.C. § 1395w-22(g)(1).

[14] Medicare Program: Establishment of the Medicare+Choice Program, 63 *Fed. Reg.* 34968, 35042-43 (June 26, 1998).

[15] At least 15 days prior to each year's annual coordinated election period, the Secretary of Health and Human Services is required to mail to each Medicare beneficiary information comparing MA plans that are or will become available in the beneficiary's area including, to the extent available, disenrollment rates for the previous 2 years (excluding disenrollment due to death or moving outside the plan's service area). The Secretary must also mail this same information, to the extent practicable, to newly eligible Medicare beneficiaries at least 30 days prior to the beginning of the individuals' initial enrollment period under the MA program. 42 U.S.C. §§ 1395w-21(d)(2)(A), (B).

[16] Pub. L. No. 110-275, §§ 162-163, 122 Stat. 2494 (codified, as amended, at 42 U.S.C. § 1395w-22(d), (e)). CMS has also published an interim final rule to implement these statutory requirements. 73 *Fed. Reg.* 54226 (Sept. 18, 2008).

[17] PFFS plans will need to demonstrate that their networks meet criteria now applicable to other MA plans, including (1) ensuring, when medically necessary, benefits are available 24 hours a day and 7 days a week, and (2) providing access to appropriate providers, including specialists for medically necessary services. A network-based plan is defined as (1) an MA plan that is a coordinated care plan, (2) a reasonable cost reimbursement plan under section 1876 of the Social Security Act, or (3) a network-based Medical Savings Account plan. A network-based plan does not include regional PPOs that do not meet provider access standards through written contracts.

[18] Beginning in 2011, PFFS plans that are sponsored by employers or unions, however, must contract with providers as part of a network regardless of their location.

[19] Unlike other MA plan sponsors, PFFS plan sponsors are currently exempt from the requirement to have quality improvement programs and are, therefore, not required to report certain quality-related information to CMS.

[20] We analyzed beneficiaries in Medicare FFS who had both Medicare Part A and Part B. We excluded plans with certain enrollment restrictions, such as plans that restrict enrollment to members of an employer group, plans that cover only Medicare Part B services, and beneficiaries in plans who live outside the 50 states, the District of Columbia, and Puerto Rico.

[21] The nine PFFS plan sponsors in our review were Blue Cross Blue Shield of Michigan; Coventry Health Care, Inc.; Geisinger Health System; Humana, Inc.; Metropolitan Health Plan; Sterling Life Insurance Company; Universal American Corporation; University of Pittsburgh Medical Center Health Plan, Inc.; and Wellpoint, Inc. We selected the largest five PFFS plan sponsors based on enrollment in July 2007 and randomly selected three PFFS plan sponsors with enrollment that ranked between the 10th and 50th percentile among all PFFS plan sponsors. We also selected one plan sponsor that was the first to offer a PFFS plan.

[22] We excluded plans with certain enrollment restrictions and beneficiaries in plans who live outside the 50 states, the District of Columbia, and Puerto Rico.

[23] An MA contract is an agreement between CMS and an MA plan sponsor that covers one or more MA plans of the same type. For example, a contract between CMS and a plan sponsor may cover at least one PFFS plan or possibly several PFFS plans.

[24] Medicare Options Compare is available at www.medicare.gov. Beneficiaries also can call 1-800-MEDICARE and have printed information sent to them if they do not have Internet access, or contact their State Health Insurance Assistance Program for help in choosing a plan.

[25] Individuals with end-stage renal disease are not eligible to enroll in most MA plans. However, if these individuals develop the disease while enrolled in an MA plan, they may remain enrolled in their plan or change plans if their plan is terminated. 42 U.S.C. §1395w-21(a)(3)(B).

[26] MA plans do not cover hospice care, a benefit that is provided under Medicare FFS.

[27] Medicare beneficiaries enrolled in an MA Medical Savings Account plan generally may not disenroll during the open enrollment period. There are other circumstances when Medicare beneficiaries can disenroll from MA plans. For example, institutionalized Medicare beneficiaries may disenroll from MA plans and elect other plans or Medicare FFS at any time

during the year. Medicare beneficiaries may also disenroll from MA plans during special election periods as approved by CMS.

[28] We use the term medically necessary to refer to Medicare-covered services that are needed for the diagnosis and treatment of a beneficiary's medical condition and meet accepted standards of medical practice.

[29] When beneficiaries enroll in any type of MA plan, including PFFS plans, and annually thereafter, the plan sponsor is required to furnish them with certain information, including the services that are covered (when medically necessary) and the associated cost-sharing obligations.

[30] MA plan sponsors and providers are also required to furnish beneficiaries with certain written notices indicating when their coverage in inpatient facilities will end and when the plan denies coverage for a service. These notices include the *Important Message from Medicare About Your Rights, Notice of Medicare Non-Coverage, Notice of Denial of Medical Coverage,* and *Detailed Explanation of Non-Coverage*. In addition, PFFS plans may allow certain providers who render services to PFFS beneficiaries to receive up to 115 percent of the contracted payment rate and bill beneficiaries the amount that exceeds the contracted rate. In this circumstance, before rendering services, hospitals must provide PFFS beneficiaries with an estimate of the cost for which the beneficiaries will be responsible.

[31] All beneficiaries enrolled in MA plans, including PFFS plans, can file an appeal if their plan will not pay for a service that a beneficiary thinks should be covered or provided.

[32] CMS officials stated that, similar to beneficiaries in PFFS plans, beneficiaries in PPO plans receiving services from out-of-network providers that do not contact their plan in advance to determine service coverage may face unexpected costs if coverage is later denied.

[33] 70 *Fed. Reg.* 4588, 4618 (Jan. 28, 2005); 42 C.F.R. § 422.504(g).

[34] We calculated the percentage of MA beneficiaries in HMOs after excluding beneficiaries who (1) were in plans with certain enrollment restrictions (i.e., employer plans, Special Needs Plans, plans that only cover Medicare Part B services) or (2) lived outside the 50 states, the District of Columbia, and Puerto Rico.

[35] Case and disease management are designed to help coordinate and manage beneficiaries' care. Discharge planning facilitates beneficiaries' discharge from a hospital. Representatives from all nine PFFS plan sponsors we interviewed stated that they offered either case or disease management to their beneficiaries, and eight sponsors stated that they also conducted discharge planning.

[36] CMS, *Medicare Managed Care Manual*, Chapter 4, Section 150.2 (Revised June 8, 2007).

[37] CMS, *2008 operational policy for PFFS plans with prior authorization and referral requirements and 2009 PBP guidance; Additional guidance on prior notification rules*, May 29, 2008. CMS had previously issued guidance for PFFS plans on prior authorization and prenotification in its 2009 Call Letter, dated March 17, 2008.

[38] To calculate this range, we excluded 10 of 158 PFFS plans and 95 of 1,410 other MA plans that were under MA contracts with fewer than 250 beneficiaries.

[39] All PFFS beneficiaries include those individuals who remained enrolled in their plans and those who subsequently disenrolled.

[40] These results may underestimate the percentage difference in projected health care expenditures between disenrollees and beneficiaries overall in PFFS and other MA plans. See appendix I for more detail.

[41] See 42 U.S.C. § 1395w-21(d)(2)(A).

[42] Balanced Budget Act of 1997, Pub. L. No. 105-33, § 4001, 111 Stat. 251, 276-286 (1997) (adding new section 1851 to the Social Security Act) (codified, as amended, at 42 U.S.C. § 1395w-21).

[43] At least 15 days prior to each year's annual coordinated election period, the Secretary is required to mail to each Medicare beneficiary information comparing MA plans that are or will become available in the beneficiary's area including, to the extent available, disenrollment rates for the previous 2 years (excluding disenrollment due to death or moving outside the plan's service area). 42 U.S.C. § 1395w-21(d)(2)(A); *see also Gray Panthers Project Fund, et al. v. Thompson*, 273 F.Supp.2d 32 (D.D.C. 2002) (holding that the Secretary was required to comply

with statutory mandates requiring mailing of comparative information to MA beneficiaries "even if compliance is cumbersome, burdensome, or costly"). In addition, the Secretary must mail these disenrollment rates, to the extent practicable, to newly eligible Medicare beneficiaries at least 30 days prior to the beginning of the individuals' initial enrollment period under the MA program. 42 U.S.C. § 1395w-21(d)(2)(B).

44 MA plan sponsors must provide, on an annual basis, the information necessary to enable CMS to provide current and potential Medicare beneficiaries the information they need to make informed decisions with respect to available choices for Medicare coverage. See 42 U.S.C. § 1395w-21(d)(7), see also 42 C.F.R. § 422.64. In addition, as required under the contract between CMS and MA plan sponsors, plan sponsors specifically must provide to CMS disenrollment rates for Medicare beneficiaries for the previous 2 years. 42 C.F.R. § 422.504(f)(2).

45 See GAO, *Medicare: Many HMOs Experience High Rates of Beneficiary Disenrollment*, GAO/HEHS-98-142 (Washington, D.C.: Apr. 30, 1998); and *Medicare: HCFA Should Release Data to Aid Consumers, Prompt Better HMO Performance*, GAO/HEHS-97-23 (Washington, D.C.: Oct. 22, 1996).

46 These risk scores were calculated for beneficiaries enrolled in July of that year and were normalized so that the average risk score for Medicare FFS beneficiaries was approximately 1.00.

47 We did not include the 2,223 beneficiaries in Medical Savings Account plans as of April 2007 in our analysis because these plans operate differently from other MA plan types. Beneficiaries in a Medical Savings Account plan receive annual deposits from CMS into an interest-bearing account to help them cover their health care costs until they have reached their plan's deductible, after which the plan is responsible for all Medicare-covered costs.

48 We analyzed beneficiaries in Medicare FFS who had both Part A and Part B.

49 We defined urban areas as those areas that are either classified as Metropolitan Statistical Areas or Micropolitan Statistical Areas. Metropolitan Statistical Areas have at least one urbanized area with a population of 50,000 or more, plus adjacent territory that has a high degree of social and economic integration with the core as measured by commuting ties. Micropolitan Statistical Areas have at least one urban cluster with a population of at least 10,000 but less than 50,000, plus adjacent territory that has a high degree of social and economic integration with the core as measured by commuting ties. We defined rural areas as those that are neither Metropolitan Statistical nor Micropolitan Statistical Areas and are not unknown.

50 The nine PFFS plan sponsors in our review were Blue Cross Blue Shield of Michigan; Coventry Health Care, Inc.; Geisinger Health System; Humana, Inc.; Metropolitan Health Plan; Sterling Life Insurance Company; Universal American Corporation; University of Pittsburgh Medical Center Health Plan, Inc.; and Wellpoint, Inc. We selected the largest five PFFS plan sponsors based on enrollment in July 2007 and randomly selected three PFFS plan sponsors with enrollment that ranked between the 10th and 50th percentile among all PFFS plan sponsors. We also selected one plan sponsor that was the first to offer a PFFS plan.

51 An MA contract is an agreement between CMS and an MA plan sponsor that covers one or more MA plans of the same type. For example, a contract between CMS and a plan sponsor may cover at least one PFFS plan or possibly several PFFS plans.

52 When calculating disenrollment rates for PFFS and other MA plans overall, we divided the total number of disenrollees by total enrollment in these plans.

53 The number of beneficiaries in these plans includes 8,918 beneficiaries in PFFS plans and 79,827 beneficiaries in other MA plans who disenrolled involuntarily and were not included in the calculation of disenrollment rates.

54 This official noted that the decline in a plan's risk score over the course of a year occurs because plans generally have a higher proportion of new Medicare beneficiaries (i.e., beneficiaries age 65 to 67 who have relatively low risk scores) at the end of the year and some older beneficiaries die who have relatively high risk scores. A plan's risk score, according to a CMS official, can

decrease from, for example, 1.00 for beneficiaries in the plan in January to 0.95 for beneficiaries in the plan in December.

[55] Medicare Options Compare is available at www.medicare.gov. Beneficiaries can also call 1-800-MEDICARE and have printed information sent to them if they do not have Internet access, or contact their State Health Insurance Assistance Program for help in choosing a plan.

In: Medicare Advantage: The Alternate Medicare … ISBN: 978-1-60876-031-2
Editors: Charles V. Baylis, pp.87-131

Chapter 3

Medicare Advantage: Increased Spending Relative to Medicare Fee-for-Service May Not Always Reduce Beneficiary Out-of-Pocket Costs

United States Government Accountability Office

Why GAO Did This Study

In 2006, the federal government spent about $59 billion on Medicare Advantage (MA) plans, an alternative to the original Medicare fee-for-service (FFS) program. Although health plans were originally envisioned in the 1980s as a potential source of Medicare savings, such plans have generally increased program spending. Payments to MA plans have been estimated to be 12 percent greater than what Medicare would have spent in 2006 had MA beneficiaries been enrolled in Medicare FFS. Some policymakers are concerned about the cost of the MA program and its contribution to overall spending on the Medicare program, which already faces serious long-term financial challenges.

MA plans receive a per member per month (PMPM) payment to provide services covered under Medicare FFS. Almost all MA plans receive an additional Medicare payment, known as a rebate. Plans use rebates and sometimes additional beneficiary premiums to fund benefits not covered under Medicare FFS, reduce premiums, or reduce beneficiary cost sharing.

This report examines for 2007 (1) MA plans' projected rebate allocations; (2) additional benefits MA plans commonly covered and their costs; (3) MA plans' projected cost sharing; and (4) MA plans' allocation of projected revenues and expenses. GAO analyzed data on MA plans' projected revenues and covered benefits for the most common types of MA plans, accounting for 71 percent of all beneficiaries in MA plans.

WHAT GAO FOUND

In 2007, plans projected that relatively little of their rebates would be spent on additional benefits compared to cost-sharing and premium reductions. Of the average projected rebate amount of $87 PMPM, plans projected they would allocate about $10 PMPM (11 percent) to additional benefits, about $61 PMPM (69 percent) to reduced cost sharing, and about $17 PMPM (20 percent) to reduced premiums.

Using funding from both rebates and additional premiums, plans covered a variety of additional benefits not covered by Medicare FFS in 2007, including dental and vision benefits. On the basis of plans' projections, GAO estimated that rebates would pay for approximately 77 percent of additional benefits and additional beneficiary premiums would pay for the remaining 23 percent.

MA plans projected that, on average, beneficiaries in their plans would have lower cost sharing than Medicare FFS cost-sharing estimates, although some MA plans projected that their beneficiaries would have higher cost sharing for certain service categories, such as home health care and inpatient services. Because cost sharing was projected to be higher for some categories of services, beneficiaries who frequently used these services could have had overall cost sharing that would be higher than under Medicare FFS.

On average, MA plans projected that they would allocate about 87 percent of total revenue ($683 of $783 PMPM) to medical expenses; approximately 9 percent ($71 PMPM) to non-medical expenses, including administration, marketing, and sales; and approximately 4 percent ($30 PMPM) to the plans' margin, sometimes called the plans' profit. About 30 percent of beneficiaries were enrolled in plans that projected they would allocate less than 85 percent of their revenues to medical expenses.

Whether the value that MA beneficiaries receive in the form of reduced cost sharing, lower premiums, and additional benefits is worth the additional cost is a decision for policymakers. However, if the policy objective is to subsidize health care costs of low-income Medicare beneficiaries, it may be more efficient to directly target subsidies to a defined low-income population than to subsidize premiums and cost sharing for all MA beneficiaries, including those who are well off. As Congress considers the design and cost of MA, it will be important for policymakers to balance the needs of beneficiaries and the necessity of addressing Medicare's long-term financial health.

In commenting on a draft of this report, the Centers for Medicare & Medicaid Services expressed concern that the report was not balanced because it did not sufficiently focus on the advantages of MA plans. GAO disagrees. This report provides information on how plans projected they would use rebates and identified instances in which MA beneficiaries could have out-of-pocket costs higher than they would have experienced under Medicare FFS.

ABBREVIATIONS

AHIP	America's Health Insurance Plans
CHAMP Act	Children's Health and Medicare Protection Act of 2007
CMS	Centers for Medicare & Medicaid Services
FFS	fee-for-service
HMO	Health Maintenance Organization
MA	Medicare Advantage
MedPAC	Medicare Payment Advisory Commission
MMA	Medicare Prescription Drug, Improvement, and Modernization Act of 2003
MSA	Medical Savings Account
PFFS	Private Fee-for-Service
PMPM	per member per month
PPO	Preferred Provider Organization
PSO	Provider-Sponsored Organization
SNP	Special Needs Plan

February 22, 2008

Congressional Requesters

In 2006, the federal government spent an estimated $59 billion on the Medicare Advantage (MA) program, an alternative to the original Medicare fee-for-service (FFS) program.[1] The MA program provides health care coverage to Medicare beneficiaries through private health plans, referred to as MA plans. As of August 2007, 8.1 million people—about one out of every five Medicare beneficiaries—were enrolled in an MA plan. Although private health plans were originally envisioned in the 1980s as a potential source of Medicare savings, such plans have generally increased overall program spending. Medicare spending on private health plans has increased rapidly since the enactment of the Medicare Prescription Drug, Improvement, and Modernization Act of 2003 (MMA),[2] rising 64 percent from 2004 to 2006, while enrollment has increased by more than 50 percent. The MMA increased payment rates for private health plans and allowed for larger annual rate increases, among other things.[3] These payment increases enabled MA plans to spend more money on additional benefits relative to those available under Medicare FFS, such as vision and hearing coverage; reductions in cost sharing—the amount a beneficiary pays for covered services; and reductions in the premiums that many Medicare FFS beneficiaries pay for coverage of outpatient services and outpatient drugs. Beginning in 2006, MA plans were required to submit bids for providing Medicare-covered services. MA plans that submitted bids below predetermined benchmarks received additional payments, known as rebates, and were required to spend their rebates on additional benefits, reduced cost sharing, reduced premiums, or a combination of the three.

As the MA program has grown, some policymakers and congressional advisors have raised concerns about the design and cost of the program as well as its effect on overall Medicare spending. The Medicare Payment Advisory Commission (MedPAC) found that payments to MA plans in 2006 exceeded by 12 percent what Medicare would have paid had MA beneficiaries received services through Medicare FFS.[4] The Congressional Budget Office estimated that $54 billion in projected Medicare spending from 2009 through 2012 is the result of setting MA plan payments above Medicare FFS spending.[5] MA plans' payments thus place an additional financial burden on the Medicare program, which the Comptroller General and others have noted already faces serious long-term financial challenges resulting from rising health care costs and the retirement of the baby boom generation.[6] Proponents of the MA program assert that the current level of MA plan payments has allowed plans to offer valuable additional benefits and make health care services more affordable for beneficiaries, particularly in rural areas where private plan options had been very limited. Further, they note that the MA program provides beneficiaries with private plan choices and enables them to select plans that reflect their preferences for premiums and cost sharing. They also point out that individuals with low incomes who do not qualify for other government health care coverage may receive some financial relief by enrolling in an MA plan. Critics of the current MA program suggest that if the policy objective is to subsidize the health care of individuals with low incomes, it would be more efficient to directly target subsidies to a well-defined low-income population instead of subsidizing the health care costs of all MA beneficiaries. Program critics also assert that a large portion of the additional payments to MA plans goes to profit and administrative costs and that some MA beneficiaries face higher cost sharing than they would if they received coverage through Medicare FFS. Questions have also been raised that while the MA program provides beneficiaries with many health plan choices, it can be difficult for even a sophisticated buyer to understand the implications of different cost-sharing arrangements. In addition, some policymakers are concerned that because premiums paid by beneficiaries in Medicare FFS are tied to both Medicare FFS and MA program spending, the excess payments to MA plans result in higher premiums for all Medicare beneficiaries.

Medicare pays MA plans a per member per month (PMPM) amount that is based on a plan's bid—its projection of the revenue it requires to provide a beneficiary with services that are covered under Medicare FFS, and a benchmark—the maximum amount Medicare will pay the plan to serve an average beneficiary. Benchmarks vary by county, and in 2007, every county in the United States had a benchmark that was at least as high as average Medicare FFS spending PMPM in that county. If the plan's bid is higher than the benchmark, Medicare pays the plan the amount of the benchmark, and the plan must charge beneficiaries a premium to collect the amount by which the bid exceeds the benchmark.[7] If the plan's bid is lower than the benchmark, Medicare pays the plan the amount of the bid and makes an additional rebate payment to the plan equal to 75 percent of the difference between the benchmark and the bid. Plans use the rebate to provide their beneficiaries with additional benefits beyond those offered in Medicare FFS, reduce premiums, reduce cost sharing, or any combination of the three. In 2007, the total amount of rebates paid to MA plans was about $8.3 billion. (See app. I for more information about how rebates are calculated.) Regardless of whether a plan's bid is above or below the benchmark, a plan may charge its beneficiaries an additional premium to provide additional benefits or reductions in cost sharing that are not otherwise financed by rebates.[8]

Given the additional spending—including rebates—for the MA program, you asked that we undertake a study on MA plans' rebates, benefit packages, and revenues. This report examines for 2007 (1) how MA plans projected they would allocate the rebates they receive, (2) what additional benefits MA plans commonly covered with the rebates and additional premiums and the projected costs of these additional benefits, (3) how MA plans' projected beneficiary cost sharing overall and by type of service compared to Medicare FFS, and (4) how MA plans projected they would allocate their revenue to medical and other expenses.

We used two primary data sources in our analyses, the 2007 Bid Pricing Tool data and the 2007 Plan Benefit Package data that MA plans submitted to the Centers for Medicare & Medicaid Services (CMS), the agency that administers Medicare. The bid pricing data contain MA plans' projections of their revenue requirements and revenue sources. Specifically, the bid pricing data contain information on the amount of rebates and additional premiums plans project they will require to fund additional benefits, reduced premiums, and reduced cost sharing. The bid pricing data also contain information about how plans' projected cost sharing compared to estimates of cost sharing in Medicare FFS and plans' projections of revenue requirements—spending on medical expenses, spending on non-medical expenses (such as marketing, sales, and administration) and their margins.[9] The benefit package data contain detailed information on the benefits and cost-sharing arrangements of plans.

We analyzed bid pricing data and benefit package data from four different plan types, which together account for 98 percent of MA enrollment—including Health Maintenance Organizations (HMO), Private Fee-for-Service (PFFS) Plans, Preferred Provider Organizations (PPO), and Provider-Sponsored Organizations (PSO).[10] Because there were only 22 PSOs and enrollment in those plans was only 1 percent of total MA enrollment, we did not report results separately for PSOs, but included them in the aggregated results we reported for all MA plans. We excluded plans that have restrictions on enrollment—such as employer plans and Special Needs Plans (SNP)—and bids for plans that only cover certain Medicare FFS services.[11] We also excluded plans with service areas that are exclusively outside the 50 states and the District of Columbia. After all exclusions, we had 2,055 plans in our study that accounted for 71 percent of all beneficiaries in MA plans. Unless otherwise noted, the analyses were based on these 2,055 plans and their beneficiaries. To address our study questions, we did the following:

- To determine how plans projected they would allocate the rebates they receive, we used the bid pricing data. We applied the proportion of the combined rebate and additional premium allocated to additional benefits, reduced premiums, and reduced cost sharing to the projected total. We restricted this analysis to those plans that received a rebate—1,874 of the 2,055 plans.

- To identify the additional benefits MA plans commonly covered with rebates and additional premiums, and the projected costs of these additional benefits, we analyzed both the benefit package and bid pricing data. We used the benefit package data to identify the additional benefits plans covered and used the bid pricing data to identify the projected cost of these additional benefits. When we analyzed the projected cost of additional benefits, we included both the rebate payments and additional premiums. We included rebates and additional premiums, rather than solely considering the effects of rebates, because rebates and premiums together fund the additional benefits that MA beneficiaries will receive. If we had estimated the cost of additional benefits funded only by the rebates, that amount would have been lower than the amount we report.
- To compare projected beneficiary cost sharing in the MA and Medicare FFS programs, we used both the bid pricing and the benefit package data. We used the bid pricing data to quantify the projected cost-sharing reduction, using the plans projections of the average cost-sharing expenditure on a PMPM basis, and compared this to CMS estimates of what the average PMPM cost-sharing expenditure would be in Medicare FFS. To obtain details on the specific cost-sharing arrangements used by the plans, we used the benefit package data. As was the case for our analysis of additional benefits, the amounts we reported for average PMPM cost sharing and cost-sharing reductions were based on the amounts projected by the plans and included funding from both rebates and additional premiums. If we had estimated the amount of cost sharing funded only by the rebates, the PMPM cost-sharing amounts would have been higher and the cost-sharing reduction amounts would have been lower.
- To identify how plans projected they would allocate their revenue to medical and other expenses, we used the bid pricing data.

Throughout the report, dollar amounts are adjusted to reflect a beneficiary of average health status. Where noted, we used August 2007 MA plan enrollment numbers to weight our results.

To determine the reliability of the bid pricing, benefits, and enrollment data, we spoke with CMS officials about the strengths and limitations of these data sets. We also conducted logic tests to ensure that the bid pricing data were reasonable and consistent, and compared the bid pricing and benefits data to ensure consistency, where applicable, across the data sets. In some cases, there were discrepancies between the two data sources. For example, some plans indicated that they had an additional benefit in the benefit package data, but did not price that additional benefit in the bid pricing data. CMS officials indicated that these discrepancies could be due, in part, to the different purposes of the benefit package and bid pricing data sets, and resulting different benefit categorizations. CMS officials said discrepancies may also be the result of some plans with low projected amounts for additional benefits categorizing those benefits as Medicare-covered services, or the bid pricing data may accurately reflect low projected prices that round to zero. In general, based on CMS's recommendations, we used the benefit package data as the most reliable data source for identifying specific benefits covered by plans, and used the bid pricing data to identify costs. We determined that the data used were sufficiently reliable for the purposes of this report. However, verifying that the projections presented in the bid pricing data actually reflect plan revenues and expenditures was beyond the scope of our work. See appendix II for more details on our scope and methodology. We conducted our work from April 2007 through February 2008 in accordance with generally accepted government auditing standards.

Results in Brief

In 2007, MA plans that received rebates projected that relatively little of the rebates would be spent on additional benefits compared to cost-sharing and premium reductions. Of the average projected rebate amount of $87 PMPM, plans projected that they would allocate about $10 PMPM (11 percent) to additional benefits, about $61 PMPM (69 percent) to reduced cost sharing, and about $17 PMPM (20 percent) to reduced premiums.

Using funding from rebates, additional premiums, or both, plans covered a variety of additional benefits in 2007, including dental, hearing, and vision benefits. The average projected PMPM costs of specific additional benefits across all MA plans ranged from $0.11 PMPM for international outpatient emergency services to $4 PMPM for dental care. On the basis of plans' projections, we estimated that rebates would pay for approximately 77 percent of these additional benefits, and additional beneficiary premiums would pay for the remaining 23 percent.

MA plans projected that, on average, beneficiaries in their plans would pay less in cost sharing than what their cost sharing would be in the Medicare FFS program, although some MA plans projected that their beneficiaries would have higher cost sharing for certain service categories. For example, 19 percent of MA beneficiaries were in plans that projected higher cost sharing for home health services and 16 percent of beneficiaries were in plans that projected higher cost sharing for inpatient services. Because cost sharing was projected to be higher for some categories of services, beneficiaries who frequently used these services could have had overall cost sharing that would be higher than under Medicare FFS. Similar to payments for additional services, we estimated that rebates would pay for about 77 percent of the cost-sharing reduction and the remainder would be paid for with additional beneficiary premiums.

Plans' total revenues in 2007 were $783 PMPM, on average, of which plans projected they would allocate approximately 87 percent ($683 PMPM) to medical expenses—referred to as a medical loss ratio of 0.87. In addition, they projected that they would allocate approximately 9 percent of total revenue ($71 PMPM) to non-medical expenses, and approximately 4 percent ($30 PMPM) to the plans' margin—sometimes called a profit. About 30 percent of beneficiaries were enrolled in plans with a medical loss ratio of less than 0.85.

Medicare spends more per beneficiary in the MA program than it does for beneficiaries in Medicare FFS, at an estimated additional cost to Medicare of $54 billion from 2009 through 2012. MA beneficiaries generally, but not always, receive additional value in the form of reduced cost sharing, lower premiums, and extra benefits, compared to Medicare FFS beneficiaries. Whether the additional value that MA beneficiaries receive is worth the additional cost to Medicare FFS beneficiaries and other taxpayers is a decision for policymakers. If the policy objective is to subsidize health care costs of low-income Medicare beneficiaries, it may be more efficient to directly target subsidies to a defined low-income population than to subsidize premiums and cost sharing for all MA beneficiaries, including those who are well off. As Congress considers the design and cost of the MA program, it will be important for policymakers to balance the needs of MA beneficiaries and Medicare FFS beneficiaries with the necessity of addressing Medicare's long-term financial health.

In commenting on a draft of this report, CMS stated that we did not consider that the majority of MA benefit packages in 2007 were better than Medicare FFS and expressed concern that the report was not balanced because it did not sufficiently focus on the advantages of MA plans. They also noted that while they did not disagree with our finding that some beneficiaries in MA plans could have higher out-of-pocket costs, we did not recognize certain factors that would have mitigated the impact of the finding. We disagree with CMS. Specifically, we recognized in the report that, on average, plans projected MA beneficiary cost sharing that was 42 percent of estimated cost sharing in Medicare FFS. Our report provides an assessment of how MA plans projected they would use their rebates in 2007, and identified important issues related to cost sharing. America's Health Insurance Plans (AHIP) indicated that they agreed with our methodology, but raised certain points that they thought the report should have made or emphasized. We added these points to the report as appropriate.

BACKGROUND

MA plans are required to cover benefits that are covered under the Medicare FFS program.[12] Medicare FFS consists of Part A; hospital insurance—which covers inpatient stays, care in skilled nursing facilities, hospice care, and some home health care, and Part B, which covers certain physician, outpatient hospital, and laboratory services, among other services. Persons aged 65 and older who meet Medicare's work requirement, certain individuals with disabilities, and most individuals with end-stage renal disease receive coverage for Part A services and pay no premium.[13] Individuals eligible for Part A can also enroll in Part B, although they are charged a Part B premium.[14] For 2007, the monthly Part B premium was set at $93.50, although high-income beneficiaries paid more. Most Medicare beneficiaries who are eligible for Medicare FFS can choose to enroll in the MA program instead of Medicare FFS.[15] MA plans operate under Medicare Part C.

All Medicare beneficiaries, regardless of their source of coverage, can choose to receive prescription drug coverage through Medicare Part D. Medicare FFS beneficiaries can enroll in stand-alone prescription drug plans, which are operated by private plan sponsors, and they generally must pay a premium to receive Part D coverage. MA beneficiaries who opt for prescription drug coverage generally receive that coverage through their MA plans, which may or may not charge an additional premium for Part D coverage. Beneficiaries enrolled in a PFFS plan that does not offer Part D coverage are allowed to enroll in a stand-alone prescription drug plan.

Beneficiaries in both Medicare FFS and MA face cost-sharing requirements for medical services. Cost sharing gives beneficiaries a financial incentive to be mindful of the costs associated with using services. Medicare FFS cost sharing takes different forms. It includes both a Part A and a Part B deductible, which is the amount a beneficiary pays for services before Medicare FFS begins to pay. For 2007, Medicare FFS required a deductible payment of $992 before it began paying for an inpatient stay, and $131 before it began paying for any Part B services. Cost sharing also includes coinsurance—a percentage payment for a given service that a beneficiary must pay, such as 20 percent of the total payment for physician visits, and copayments—a standard amount a beneficiary must pay for a medical service, such as $248 per day for days 61 through 90 of an inpatient stay in 2007.

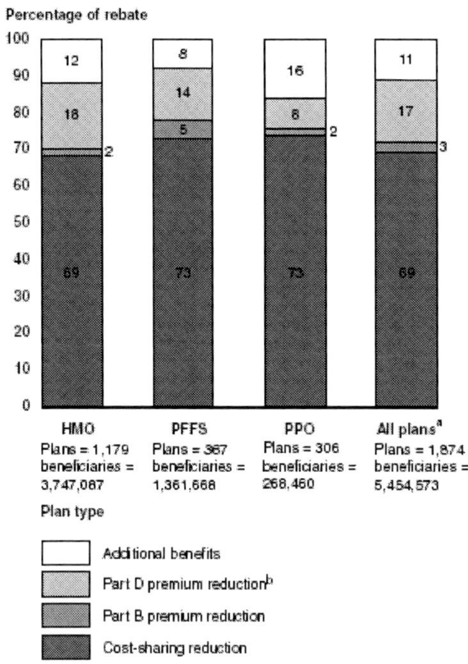

Source: GAO analysis of 2007 CMS Bid Pricing Tool data.

Notes: Percentages may not sum to 100 due to rounding. Percentages are weighted by August 2007 plan enrollment. Employer plans, Part B only plans, SNPs, regional PPOs, and plans with service areas that are exclusively outside of the 50 states and the District of Columbia were excluded from the analysis. This analysis includes only the 1,874 plans that received a rebate.

[a] The "All plans" category includes HMOs, PFFS plans, PPOs, and PSOs. Results are not reported separately for PSOs because there were only 22 PSO plans and enrollment in those plans constituted 1 percent of total MA enrollment.

[b] Of the 1,874 plans that received a rebate, 1,423 offered Part D benefits to their beneficiaries. Of those that offered Part D, 1,037 reduced Part D premiums.

Figure 1. Projected Rebate Allocation to Additional Benefits, Premium Reductions, and Cost-Sharing Reductions by Plan Type, 2007

Medicare allows MA plans to have cost-sharing requirements that are different from Medicare FFS's cost-sharing requirements. Plans may require more or less cost sharing than Medicare FFS for a given service, although, on average, a plan cannot require overall cost sharing that exceeds what beneficiaries would be expected to pay under Medicare FFS. MA plans may establish dollar limits on the amount a beneficiary spends on cost sharing in a year of coverage. In contrast, Medicare FFS has no total cost-sharing limit.[16] Plans can use both out-of-pocket maximums, limits that can apply to all services but can exclude certain service categories, and service-specific maximums, limits that apply to one service category. These limits help provide financial protection to beneficiaries who might otherwise have high cost-sharing expenses.

Table 1. Rebate Amount PMPM Allocated to Additional Benefits, Premium Reductions, and Cost-Sharing Reductions by Plan Type, 2007

	HMO Plans = 1,179 Beneficiaries = 3,747,087	**PFFS Plans = 367 Beneficiaries = 1,361,668**	**PPO Plans = 306 Beneficiaries = 268,460**	**All plans[a] Plans = 1,874 Beneficiaries = 5,454,573**
Rebate average	$93.29	$70.06	$55.26	$87.44
Amount of rebate allocated to				
Additional benefits[b]	11.36	5.58	9.08	9.95
Part D premium reduction[c]	16.35	9.51	4.51	14.70
Part B premium reduction	1.59	3.62	1.06	2.29
Cost-sharing reduction[b]	63.99	51.34	40.61	60.51

Source: GAO analysis of 2007 CMS Bid Pricing Tool data.

Notes: Values are weighted by August 2007 plan enrollment and are standardized to represent a beneficiary of average health status. Employer plans, Part B only plans, SNPs, regional PPOs, and plans with service areas that are exclusively outside of the 50 states and the District of Columbia are excluded from the analysis. This analysis included only the 1,874 plans that received a rebate.

[a] The "All plans" category includes HMOs, PFFS plans, PPOs, and PSOs. Results are not reported separately for PSOs because there were only 22 PSO plans and enrollment in those plans constituted 1 percent of total MA enrollment.

[b] The rebate amounts allocated to cost sharing and additional benefits included some non-medical expenses, such as administrative costs and plans' margins.

[c] Of the 1,874 plans that received a rebate, 1,423 offered Part D benefits to their beneficiaries. Of those that offered Part D, 1,037 reduced Part D premiums.

CMS officials said that they evaluate the cost-sharing arrangements of MA plans to determine if cost sharing is too high for services likely to be used by a beneficiary with below average health status. According to CMS officials, in 2007, if an MA plan (1) had no out-of-pocket maximum, (2) had an out-of-pocket maximum above $3,100, or (3) had an out-of-pocket maximum of $3,100 or below and excluded certain categories of service from that maximum, CMS compared the plan's cost sharing for certain service categories to thresholds that CMS based on Medicare FFS cost-sharing levels.[17] If a plan exceeded one or more thresholds, CMS may have sought to negotiate with the plan over its cost sharing. According to CMS officials, the decision to negotiate was based on various factors, including the extent to which the thresholds were exceeded, local market comparisons, and the extent to which high cost sharing in one category was balanced with low cost sharing in another.[18]

MA Plans Projected That They Would Allocate Relatively Little of Their Rebates to Additional Benefits and the Majority to Reduced Cost Sharing

MA plans that received rebates projected, on average, that their rebates would be $87 PMPM. The plans projected that they would allocate a relatively small amount to additional benefits, compared to cost-sharing and premium reductions. Plans projected that, on average, about 11 percent of their rebates would be allocated to additional benefits, 69 percent to reduced cost sharing, 17 percent to Part D premium reductions, and 3 percent to Part B premium reductions. The average projected rebate allocation to additional benefits and reduced premiums varied by plan type. For example, PPOs projected that they would allocate less to Part D premium reductions and more to additional benefits than other plan types. PFFS plans projected that they would allocate less to additional benefits than other plan types. (See figure 1.)

In dollar terms, the average projected rebates varied by plan type, from $55 PMPM for PPOs to $93 PMPM for HMOs. The dollar portions of the rebates that plans allocated to cost sharing varied, reflecting the variation in the average amount of the rebate. For example, on average, both PFFS plans and PPOs projected that they would allocate 73 percent of their rebate to cost-sharing reductions, but PFFS plans projected this would average $51 PMPM while PPOs projected this would average $41 PMPM.[19] (See table 1.) For more information on the variation in how plans allocated rebates and the rebate amounts, see appendix III.

Table 2. Percentage of Beneficiaries in Plans That Charge an Additional Premium and Average Amount of Additional Premium by Plan Type, 2007

	HMO **Plans = 1,209** **Beneficiaries = 3,977,161**	**PFFS** **Plans = 479** **Beneficiaries = 1,408,103**	**PPO** **Plans = 345** **Beneficiaries = 301,746**	**All plans[a]** **Plans = 2,055** **Beneficiaries = 5,764,368**
Percentage of beneficiaries in plans that charge an additional premium and do not receive a rebate	6	3	11	5
Percentage of beneficiaries in plans that charge an additional premium and receive a rebate	36	28	72	35
Average amount of additional premium (PMPM)	$61.87	$42.09	$60.47	$58.00

Source: GAO analysis of 2007 CMS Bid Pricing Tool data.

Notes: Values are weighted by August 2007 plan enrollment and are standardized to represent a beneficiary of average health status. Employer plans, Part B only plans, SNPs, regional PPOs, and plans with service areas that are exclusively outside of the 50 states and the District of Columbia were excluded from the analysis.

[a] The "All plans" category includes HMOs, PFFS plans, PPOs, and PSOs. Results are not reported separately for PSOs because there were only 22 PSO plans and enrollment in those plans constituted 1 percent of total MA enrollment.

While nearly all MA enrollees were in plans that received rebates, some plans charged additional premiums either in addition to the rebate or as the sole funding source to pay for additional benefits, reduced cost sharing, or a combination of the two. In 2007, approximately 41 percent of beneficiaries (about 2.3 million people) were enrolled in an MA plan that charged an additional premium. There were differences in the extent to which plans charged additional premiums by plan type. For example, 31 percent of beneficiaries enrolled in PFFS plans were charged an additional premium, compared to 83 percent of beneficiaries enrolled in PPOs. Of plans that charged an additional premium, the average additional premium was $58 PMPM.[20] (See table 2.) Plans that received rebates and charged additional premiums had lower rebates ($54 PMPM on average), than plans that received rebates and did not charge an additional premium ($107 PMPM on average), and these plans allocated less of their rebates to premium reductions and more to additional benefits and cost-sharing reductions.[21]

MA Plans Used Rebates and Additional Premiums to Cover Additional Benefits Such as Dental, Hearing, and Vision

MA Plans Used Rebates and Additional Premiums to Cover Additional Benefits Such as Dental, Hearing, and Vision MA plans covered several common additional benefits with the rebates, additional premiums, or both. These benefits included

- dental benefits, which may include oral exams, teeth cleanings, fluoride treatments, dental X-rays, or emergency dental services;
- health education benefits, which may include nutritional training, smoking cessation, health club memberships, or nursing hotlines;
- hearing benefits, which may include coverage for hearing tests, hearing aid fittings, and hearing aid evaluations;
- inpatient facility stays, which may include additional inpatient facility days beyond those covered under Medicare FFS;
- international coverage for outpatient emergency services;
- skilled nursing facility stays, which include days in a skilled nursing facility beyond those covered under Medicare FFS; and
- vision benefits, which may include coverage for routine eye exams, contacts, or eyeglasses (lenses and frames).

Almost all plans covered international outpatient emergency services and additional days in a skilled nursing facility and inpatient facility beyond what Medicare FFS covers. The percentage of plans covering dental, vision, or hearing services varied by plan type. For example, PFFS plans were more likely to cover hearing and less likely to cover dental and vision services than HMOs and PPOs. (See figure 2.)

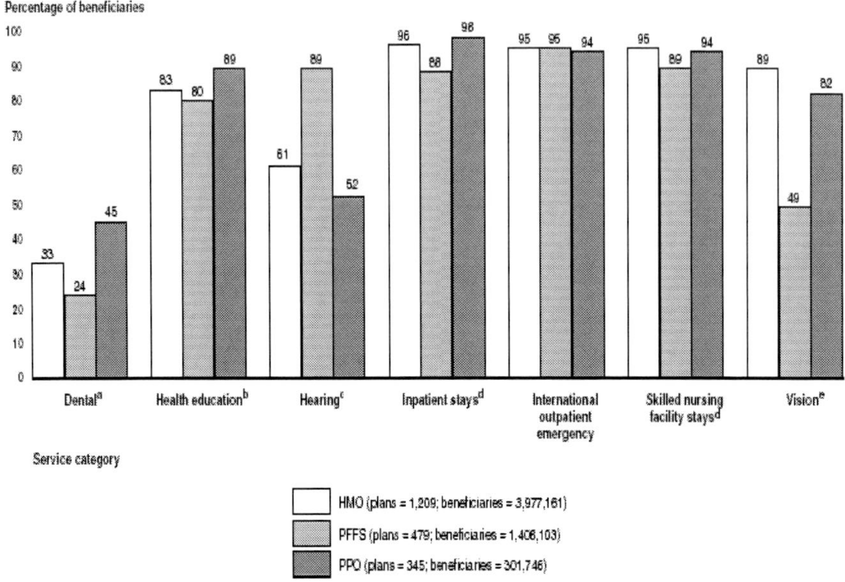

Source: GAO analysis of 2007 CMS Bid Pricing Tool data.

Notes: The percentages of beneficiaries in plans that have additional benefits are as of August 2007. This analysis included additional benefits funded by both rebates and additional premiums. Employer plans, Part B only plans, SNPs, regional PPOs, and plans with service areas that are exclusively outside of the 50 states and the District of Columbia were excluded from the analysis.

[a] Dental benefits may include oral exams, teeth cleanings, fluoride treatments, dental X-rays, or emergency dental services.

[b] Health education benefits may include nutritional training, smoking cessation, health club memberships, or nursing hotlines.

[c] Hearing benefits may include coverage for hearing tests, hearing aid fittings, and hearing aid evaluations.

[d] Inpatient stays and skilled nursing facility stays may include additional days beyond what Medicare FFS covers.

[e] Vision benefits may include coverage for routine eye exams, contacts, or eyeglasses (lenses and frames).

Figure 2. Percentage of Beneficiaries in Plans Covering Additional Benefits by Plan Type, 2007

Table 3. Average Projected PMPM Costs of Additional Benefits by Service Category and Plan Type for Plans That Offered Benefits and Reported Costs, 2007

	HMO		PFFS		PPO		All plans[a]	
	Number of plans	Average cost (PMPM)	Number of plans	Average cost (PMPM)	Number of plans	Average cost (PMPM)	Number of plans	Average cost (PMPM)
Dental[b]	435	$3.72	29	$4.34	80	$5.79	555	$4.00
Health education[c]	641	2.01	97	1.12	165	1.95	920	1.88
Hearing[d]	865	0.86	185	0.97	235	1.51	1301	0.92
Inpatient stays[e]	966	1.74	255	1.31	240	1.75	1482	1.69
International outpatient emergency	698	0.13	165	0.05	204	0.06	1083	0.11
Skilled nursing facility stays[e]	576	1.33	119	0.38	94	1.55	801	1.14
Vision[f]	1,076	3.41	182	2.37	280	5.76	1559	3.37

Source: GAO analysis of 2007 CMS Bid Pricing Tool data.

Notes: Dollar amounts are weighted by August 2007 plan enrollment and are standardized to represent a beneficiary of average health status. We considered an MA plan to have covered an additional benefit if it projected that it would allocate at least $.01 PMPM of revenue to the additional benefit. Employer plans, Part B only plans, SNPs, regional PPOs, and plans with service areas that are exclusively outside of the 50 states and the District of Columbia were excluded from the analysis.

[a] The "All plans" category includes HMOs, PFFS plans, PPOs, and PSOs. Results are not reported separately for PSOs because there are only 22 PSO plans and enrollment in those plans constituted 1 percent of total MA enrollment.

[b] Dental benefits may include oral exams, teeth cleanings, fluoride treatments, dental X-rays, or emergency dental services.

[c] Health education benefits may include nutritional training, smoking cessation, health club memberships, or nursing hotlines.

[d] Hearing benefits may include coverage for hearing tests, hearing aid fittings, and hearing aid evaluations.

[e] Inpatient stays and skilled nursing facility stays may include additional days beyond what Medicare FFS covers.

[f] Vision benefits may include coverage for routine eye exams, contacts, or eyeglasses (lenses and frames).

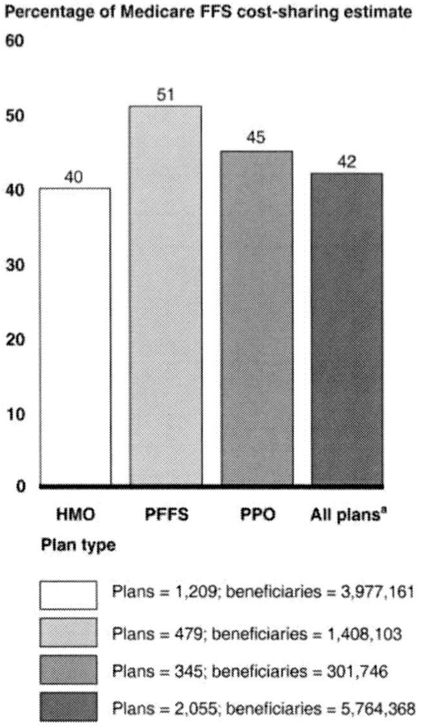

Source: GAO analysis of 2007 CMS Bid Pricing Tool data.

Notes: Employer plans, Part B only plans, SNPs, regional PPOs, and plans with service areas that are exclusively outside of the 50 states and the District of Columbia were excluded from the analysis. Numbers are weighted by August 2007 plan enrollment.

[a] The "All plans" category includes HMOs, PFFS plans, PPOs, and PSOs. Results are not reported separately for PSOs because there were only 22 PSO plans and enrollment in those plans constituted 1 percent of total MA enrollment.

Figure 3. Average Projected Cost Sharing for MA Beneficiaries Compared to Their Cost Sharing in Medicare FFS, by Plan Type, 2007

The average projected dollar amount of the common additional benefits across all MA plans ranged from $0.11 PMPM for international outpatient emergency services to $4 PMPM for dental care. These estimates were based on the subset of plans that provided cost projections in the categories associated with the benefits. The number of plans included in the averages varies from the number of plans offering the benefits in part because some plans did not consistently include the same additional services in the same benefit categories. For example, some plans categorized all or part of the costs associated with additional vision benefits in other categories, such as professional services.[22] These estimates are also based on plans' reported funding for additional benefits from both rebates and additional premiums. Had we limited our analysis to additional benefits funded only from rebates, the estimated amounts of the additional benefits would have been lower. On the basis of plan projections, we estimated that rebates would pay for most of the additional benefits plans provided (77 percent), while additional premiums would pay for the remainder (23 percent). Table 3 provides a summary of the projected costs of additional benefits.

MA Plans Projected That MA Beneficiaries, on Average, Would Have Lower Cost Sharing Than if They Were in Medicare FFS, but Some MA Beneficiaries Could Pay More

For 2007, MA plans projected that MA beneficiary cost sharing would be 42 percent of estimated cost sharing in Medicare FFS. (See figure 3.) Plans projected that their beneficiaries, on average, would pay $49 PMPM in cost sharing, and they estimated that Medicare FFS equivalent cost sharing for their beneficiaries was $116 PMPM. On the basis of plans' projections, we estimated that about 77 percent of the reduction in beneficiary cost sharing was funded by rebates with the remainder being funded by additional beneficiary premiums.

Although plans projected that beneficiaries' overall cost sharing was lower, on average, than Medicare FFS cost-sharing estimates, some MA plans projected that cost sharing for certain categories of services was higher than Medicare FFS cost-sharing estimates. For example, 19 percent of MA beneficiaries were enrolled in plans that projected higher cost sharing for home health services, on average, than Medicare FFS, which has no cost sharing for this service at all, and 16 percent of beneficiaries were enrolled in plans that projected higher cost sharing for inpatient services compared to Medicare FFS estimates.[23] (See table 4.) Because cost sharing is higher for some categories of services, some beneficiarics who frequently use these services can have overall cost sharing that is higher than what they would pay under Medicare FFS.

Cost sharing for particular categories of services varied substantially among MA plans. For example, we found significant variation in cost sharing for inpatient services. Some MA beneficiaries were in plans with no cost sharing for inpatient services. More than half a million MA beneficiaries, representing 9 percent of MA beneficiaries, were in 193 plans with no deductibles, copayments, or coinsurance requirements for inpatient services as of August 2007. Beneficiaries in these plans with long or frequent hospital stays could have saved thousands compared to what their cost sharing would have been if they were enrolled in Medicare FFS, which typically included a $992 deductible, a $248 daily copayment for hospital stays lasting between 61 and 90 days, and additional coinsurance payments for professional services provided in the hospital.[24]

Other MA beneficiaries, however, could have paid substantially more than Medicare FFS beneficiaries for inpatient care. We found 80 MA plans that charged a daily copayment of $200 or more for the first 10 days of a hospital admission and placed high or no limits on out-of-pocket costs for inpatient services.[25] These 80 MA plans also had more than half a million beneficiaries. Beneficiary cost sharing in these 80 plans could have been $2,000 or more for a 10-day hospital stay, and $3,000 or more for three average-length hospital stays.[26] Figure 4 provides an illustrative example of an MA plan that could have exposed a beneficiary to higher inpatient costs than under Medicare FFS. While the plan in this illustrative example had lower cost sharing than Medicare FFS for initial hospital stays of 4 days or less as well as initial hospital stays of 30 days or more, for stays of other lengths the MA plan could have cost beneficiaries more than $1,000 above out-of-pocket costs under Medicare FFS. The disparity between out-of-pocket costs under the MA plan and costs under Medicare FFS was largest when comparing additional hospital visits in the same benefit period, since Medicare FFS does not charge a deductible if an admission occurs within 60 days of a previous admission.

As of August 2007, about 48 percent of MA beneficiaries were enrolled in plans that had an out-of-pocket maximum, which helps protect beneficiaries against high spending on cost sharing.[27] (See figure 5.) Of the three most common MA plan types, beneficiaries in PFFS plans were the most likely to be in a plan with an out-of-pocket maximum, but PFFS plans also had the highest average out-of-pocket maximum. For MA plans that had an out-of-pocket maximum, the average amount was $3,463. See appendix IV for further details on out-of-pocket maximums.

An out-of-pocket maximum does not always cover all categories of services. Some MA plans excluded some services from the out-of-pocket maximum. Beneficiaries who use these excluded services may pay more in total cost sharing than is indicated by the plan's out-of-pocket maximum. Part B drugs, which include drugs that are typically physician-administered drugs, were most often excluded from the out-of-pocket maximum—29 percent of MA plans with an out-of-pocket maximum excluded some Part B drugs from that maximum.[28] (See table 5.) Plans that excluded a certain service category from the out-of-pocket maximum did not necessarily exclude all services from that category. For example, many plans excluded Part B drugs from the out-of-pocket maximum if they were obtained from a pharmacy, but according to CMS, did not exclude Part B drugs administered by a physician.

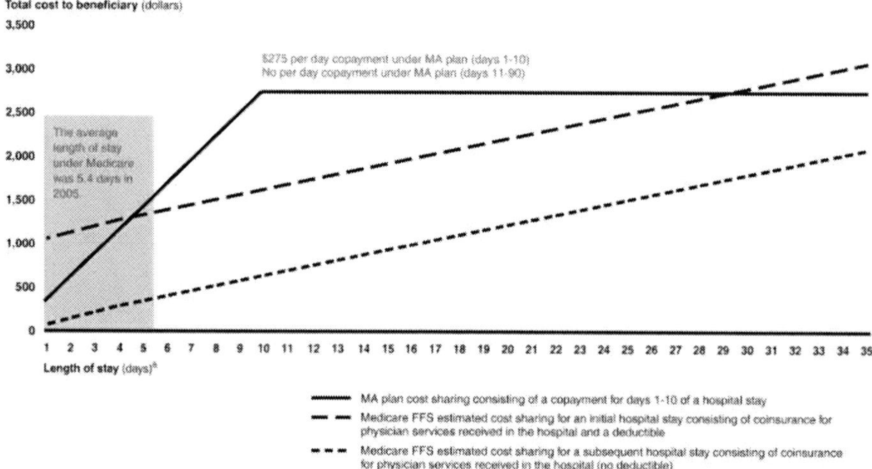

Source: GAO analysis of 2007 CMS Plan Benefit Package data and CMS actuarial data.

Notes: In this example, the MA plan charged a $275 daily copayment for the first 10 days of the hospital stay, and charged no additional copayment for days 11 through 90. The plan had a $4,000 out-of-pocket maximum. In contrast, in 2007 Medicare FFS charged a $992 deductible for an initial hospital stay in a benefit period and $248 per day for days 61 through 90 of a hospital stay. Medicare FFS beneficiaries paid no deductible for a subsequent hospital stay if it occurred within 60 days of the previous stay in an inpatient facility. In addition, Medicare FFS beneficiaries must pay coinsurance for physician services received while in the hospital. The charges associated with these physician services averaged $73 per day for the first 4 days of the hospital stay, and $58 per day for the remaining days of a hospital stay through 90 days. This example assumes that the beneficiary was charged the average coinsurance. The actual amount of coinsurance a beneficiary pays varies based on the amount of services a beneficiary receives, and charges can be above or below the average.

[a] Nearly 88 percent of hospital stays under Medicare were 10 days or less in 2004 according to CMS data. About 3 percent of hospital stays were 20 days or longer, and 1 percent of stays were longer than 30 days.

Figure 4. Example of an MA Plan with Inpatient Cost Sharing Different from the Medicare FFS Program

Table 4. Beneficiaries in MA Plans with Higher Projected Cost Sharing Than Medicare FFS for a Given Service Category by Plan Type, 2007

	HMO Plans = 1,209 Beneficiaries = 3,977,161		PFFS Plans = 479 Beneficiaries = 1,408,103		PPO Plans = 345 Beneficiaries = 301,746		All plans[a] Plans = 2,055 Beneficiaries = 5,764,368	
	Number	Percentage	Number	Percentage	Number	Percentage	Number	Percentage
Home health services[b]	422,078	11	393,523	28	253,242	84	1,069,023	19
Inpatient services[c]	699,763	18	170,737	12	66,746	22	937,246	16
Skilled nursing facility services	384,960	10	67,017	5	47,094	16	499,071	9
Durable medical equipment, prosthetics, and supplies	92,070	2	110,147	8	13,324	4	215,541	4
Part B drugs[d]	88,458	2	7,975	1	4,806	2	101,416	2
Outpatient facility services[e]	31,359	1	0	0	138	0	31,497	1
Professional services[c]	14,641	0	5,781	0	26,611	9	47,033	1

Source: GAO analysis of 2007 CMS Bid Pricing Tool data.

Notes: Employer plans, Part B only plans, SNPs, regional PPOs, and plans with service areas that are exclusively outside of the 50 states and the District of Columbia were excluded from the analysis.

[a] The "All plans" category includes HMOs, PFFS plans, PPOs, and PSOs. Results are not reported separately for PSOs because there were only 22 PSO plans and enrollment in those plans constituted 1 percent of total MA enrollment.

[b] Home health services include skilled nursing services, home health aides, and certain therapy services, all provided in the home setting.

[c] Many MA plans include cost sharing for professional services, such as physician visits received during a hospital stay, in their inpatient cost-sharing amount. As a result, the cost sharing for professional services may be understated for MA plans, while the inpatient cost sharing may be overstated for MA plans. Professional services include physician visits, therapy, and radiology, among other services.

[d] Part B drugs are drugs that are covered under Medicare Part B, and they include drugs that are typically administered by a physician. Many plans excluded Part B drugs from the out-of-pocket maximum if they were obtained from a pharmacy, but according to CMS, did not exclude Part B drugs administered by a physician.

[e] Outpatient facility services include surgery, emergency, and other services provided in an outpatient facility.

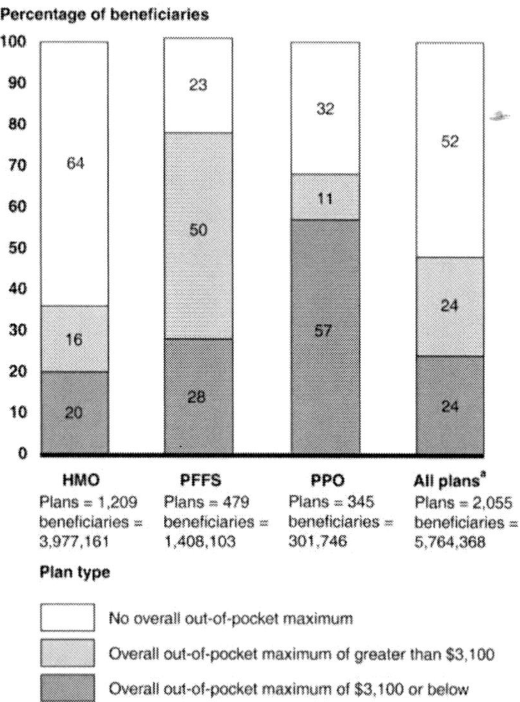

Source: GAO analysis of 2007 CMS Bid Pricing Tool data.

Notes: For 2007, CMS generally applied less stringent criteria in evaluating a plan's cost-sharing requirements if the plan had an out-of-pocket maximum of $3,100 or below. If a plan had two out-of-pocket maximums—one for in-network services and one for combined in- and out-of-network services, then we used the lower value for this analysis. Some plans without an out-of-pocket maximum did have a service-specific maximum. Twenty-one percent of plans with no out-of-pocket maximum had a service-specific maximum for inpatient acute services, and 16 percent of plans with no out-of-pocket maximum had a service-specific maximum for inpatient psychiatric services. Employer plans, Part B only plans, SNPs, regional PPOs, and plans with service areas that are exclusively outside of the 50 states and the District of Columbia were excluded from the analysis. Some numbers do not add up to 100 due to rounding.

[a] The "All plans" category includes HMOs, PFFS plans, PPOs, and PSOs. Results are not reported separately for PSOs because there were only 22 PSO plans and enrollment in those plans constituted 1 percent of total MA enrollment.

Figure 5. Beneficiaries in MA Plans by Out-of-Pocket Maximum Amount and Plan Type, 2007.

Table 5. MA Plans That Exclude Some Services under a Service Category from Their Out-of-Pocket Maximum

	Number of plans Plans = 1,016	Percentage of plans Plans = 1,016	Number of beneficiaries Beneficiaries = 2,738,531	Percentage of beneficiaries Beneficiaries = 2,738,531
Part B drugs[a]	296	29	1,107,876	40
Outpatient substance abuse	233	23	645,997	24
Physician specialist, excluding psychiatric	230	23	641,270	23
Mental health, non-physician	230	23	630,504	23
Psychiatric	218	21	602,500	22
Home health services	211	21	569,618	21
Prosthetics and medical supplies	128	13	603,952	22
Durable medical equipment	116	11	565,413	21
Outpatient hospital	72	7	192,182	7
Inpatient hospital, psychiatric	37	4	149,105	5
Skilled nursing facility	34	3	100,700	4
Inpatient hospital, acute	19	2	29,937	1

Source: GAO analysis of 2007 CMS Plan Benefit Package data.

Notes: We considered an MA plan to have an out-of-pocket maximum if the plan had either an in-network out-of-pocket maximum or an out-of-pocket maximum for both in-network and out-of-network services. A plan was considered to have excluded a service category from the out-of-pocket maximum if the out-of-pocket maximum did not cover that service category and if the plan had no service-specific maximum for that category. Plans that excluded a certain service category from the out-of-pocket maximum did not necessarily exclude all services from that category. HMOs, PFFS plans, PPOs, and PSOs were included in the analysis. Employer plans, Part B only plans, SNPs, regional PPOs, and plans with service areas that were exclusively outside of the 50 states and the District of Columbia were excluded from the analysis. Only plans with an out-of-pocket maximum were included in this analysis.

[a] Many plans excluded Part B drugs from the out-of-pocket maximum if they were obtained from a pharmacy, but according to CMS, did not exclude Part B drugs administered by a physician.

Approximately 87 Percent of Total Revenue Projected to Be Allocated to Medical Expenses, but Projections Varied among Individual Plans

For 2007, MA plans projected that of their total revenues ($783 PMPM), they would allocate approximately 87 percent ($683 PMPM) to medical expenses, resulting in an average medical loss ratio of approximately 0.87. MA plans projected that they would allocate approximately 9 percent of total revenue ($71 PMPM) to non-medical expenses, and approximately 4 percent ($30 PMPM) to the plans' margin, on average.[29]

While there was little variation in the average projected medical loss ratio by plan type, there was variation among individual plans. For example, we found that about 30 percent of beneficiaries—about 1.7 million—were enrolled in plans with a medical loss ratio of less than 0.85—the threshold included in the Children's Health and Medicare Protection Act of 2007 (CHAMP Act).[30] (See figure 6.) A CMS official we spoke to stated that the medical loss ratio may vary for reasons other than utilization and the cost of providing care. For example, some MA plans may categorize the costs of delivering care management services as a medical expense, while other plans may include this as a non-medical expense.

MA plans projected expenses separately for four distinct non-medical expense categories—marketing and sales, direct administration, indirect administration, and the net cost of private reinsurance.[31] On average, MA plans projected allocating total revenue to non-medical expenses approximately as follows:

- 2.4 percent to marketing and sales;
- 2.9 percent to direct administration, such as customer service and medical management;
- 3.7 percent to indirect administration, such as accounting operations and human resources; and
- 0.1 percent to the net cost of private reinsurance.

Of these four non-medical expense categories, the largest difference between plan types' allocation of revenue to non-medical expenses was in the category of marketing and sales. On average, as a percentage of total revenue, projected marketing and sales expenses were 2 percent ($16 PMPM) for HMOs, 3.6 percent ($27 PMPM) for PFFS plans, and 2 percent ($17 PMPM) for PPOs. (See figure 7.)

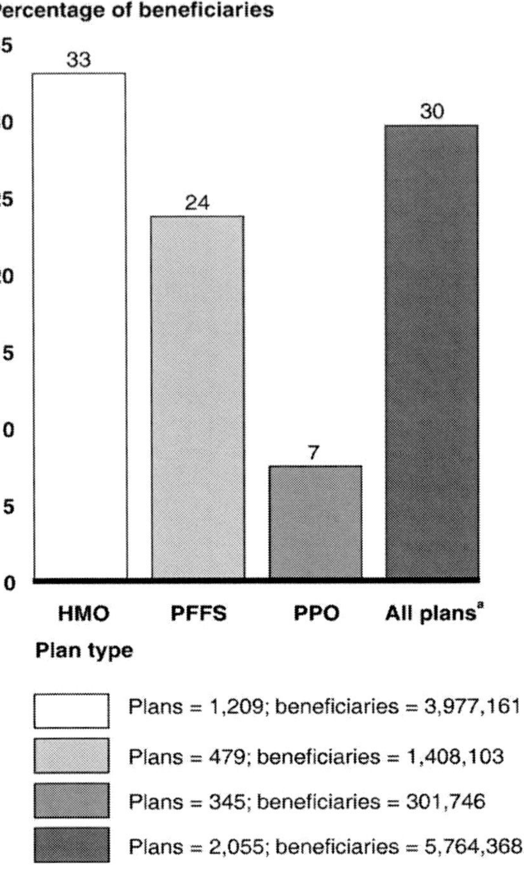

Source: GAO analysis of 2007 CMS Bid Pricing Tool data.

Notes: A CMS official indicated that the percentage of revenues allocated to medical expenses (the medical loss ratio) may vary across plans for reasons other than utilization and the cost of providing care. For example, some MA plans may categorize the costs of delivering care management services as a medical expense, while other plans may include this as a non-medical expense. Employer plans, Part B only plans, SNPs, regional PPOs, and plans with service areas that are exclusively outside of the 50 states and the District of Columbia were excluded from the analysis.

[a] The "All plans" category includes HMOs, PFFS plans, PPOs, and PSOs. Results are not reported separately for PSOs because there were only 22 PSO plans and enrollment in those plans constituted 1 percent of total MA enrollment.

Figure 6. Percentage of Beneficiaries in MA Plans That Project Allocating Less Than 85 Percent of Total Revenues to Medical Expenses, by Plan Type, 2007

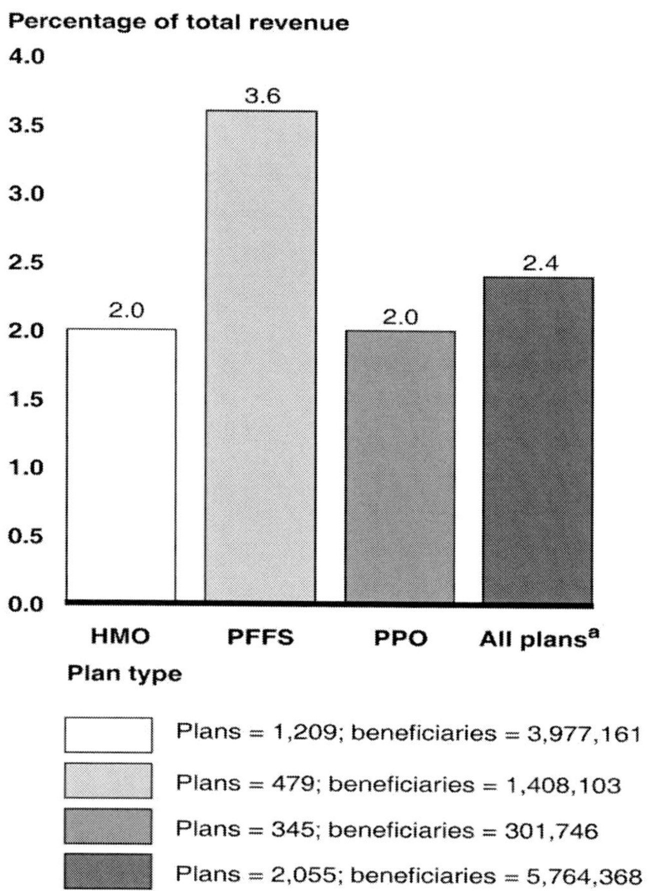

Source: GAO analysis of 2007 CMS Bid Pricing Tool data.

Notes: Percentages are weighted by August 2007 enrollment. Employer plans, Part B only plans, SNPs, regional PPOs, and plans with service areas that are exclusively outside of the 50 states and the District of Columbia were excluded from the analysis.

[a] The "All plans" category includes HMOs, PFFS plans, PPOs, and PSOs. Results are not reported separately for PSOs because there were only 22 PSO plans and enrollment in those plans constituted 1 percent of total MA enrollment.

Figure 7. MA Plans' Projected Marketing and Sales Expenses by Plan Type, 2007

Concluding Observations

Medicare spends more per beneficiary in MA than it does for beneficiaries in Medicare FFS, at an estimated additional cost to Medicare of $54 billion from 2009 through 2012. Under the current payment system, the average MA plan receives a Medicare rebate equal to approximately $87 PMPM, on average. In 2007, MA plans projected that they would use the vast majority of their rebates—approximately 89 percent—to reduce enrollees' premiums and to lower their out-of-pocket costs for Medicare-covered services. Plans projected that they would use a relatively small portion of their rebates—approximately 11 percent—to provide benefits that are not covered under Medicare FFS. Although the rebates generally have helped to make health care more affordable for many beneficiaries enrolled in MA plans, some beneficiaries may face higher expenses than they would in Medicare FFS. Further, because premiums paid by beneficiaries in Medicare FFS are tied to both Medicare FFS and MA costs, the additional payments to MA plans have increased the premiums paid by beneficiaries in Medicare FFS as well as contributed to the substantial long-term financial challenge that Medicare faces. Whether the value that MA beneficiaries receive in the form of reduced cost sharing, lower premiums, and extra benefits is worth the increased cost borne by beneficiaries in Medicare FFS and other taxpayers is a decision for policymakers. However, if the policy objective is to subsidize health care costs of low-income Medicare beneficiaries, it may be more efficient to directly target subsidies to a defined low-income population than to subsidize premiums and cost sharing for all MA beneficiaries, including those who are well off. As Congress considers the design and cost of the MA program, it will be important for policymakers to balance the needs of beneficiaries—including those in MA plans and those in Medicare FFS—with the necessity of addressing Medicare's long-term financial health.

Agency and Other External Comments and Our Evaluation

CMS provided us with written comments on a draft of this report which are reprinted in appendix V, and AHIP, a national association that represents companies providing health insurance coverage, provided us with oral comments.

CMS Comments

In general, CMS commented that the report did not recognize that the majority of MA benefit packages in 2007 were better and provided more protection for out-of-pocket costs than Medicare FFS. It stated that the report failed to acknowledge that MA plans provide beneficiaries with the ability to choose a plan that best meets individual medical and financial needs. CMS also expressed concern that the report was not balanced because it did not sufficiently focus on the advantages of MA plans. We disagree with CMS that we did not consider that most MA plans offered better cost sharing than Medicare FFS. We noted in the first paragraph of our cost sharing finding that, overall, plans projected MA beneficiary cost sharing that was 42 percent of estimated cost sharing in Medicare FFS. Regarding the absence of information about MA plans providing beneficiaries with choices, this was not the focus of our research. However, we agree the issue provides important context and therefore we noted in the report's introduction the additional choice MA plans provide Medicare beneficiaries. We disagree that the report is not balanced. We provided a fact-based assessment of how rebates were projected to be used in 2007, and identified important issues related to cost sharing. Even though cost sharing would be less, on average, in MA plans than in Medicare FFS, an important finding of our report is that beneficiaries who use certain services with high cost sharing in MA plans could have higher overall out-of-pocket costs than under Medicare FFS.

CMS provided several additional comments. CMS commented that it did not disagree with our finding that 16 percent of beneficiaries were in plans with higher inpatient cost sharing than Medicare FFS. However, it noted that our discussion of the issue and accompanying table and figure did not account for several factors that would have mitigated the impact of the finding. Specifically, CMS commented that we should have considered that MA plans generally combine physician cost sharing in the hospital with inpatient hospital cost sharing, which would have decreased the difference in cost sharing between MA plans and Medicare FFS. Although we had noted this in table notes in the draft, we agree that this should be clearer and modified our text and accompanying figure comparing MA and Medicare FFS cost sharing, and clarified existing table notes. We also modified the text and accompanying figure to differentiate between first and subsequent admissions within the same benefit period, in response to CMS comments. These changes did not affect our finding that some beneficiaries could have cost sharing that was considerably higher than in Medicare FFS.

CMS also commented that we should have discussed the mitigating impact of particularly long hospitalizations because beneficiaries with long inpatient hospitals stays in MA plans are likely to have lower cost sharing than under Medicare FFS. We acknowledged CMS's point and addressed this issue in the finding and modified the accompanying figure. However, most beneficiaries have relatively short lengths of stay. For example, in 2005, the average length for an inpatient stay was 5.4 days. This modification did not change our message that some beneficiaries in MA plans could have higher out-of-pocket costs.

In addition, CMS commented that we should have noted that many plans have "effective" out-of-pocket maximums for inpatient stays even if they are not specified as such in the plan benefit package. For example, plans may require copayments for specific days of an inpatient stay, such as days 1 through 6, but not for any days beyond the sixth day, thereby capping maximum cost sharing for the stay. We agree that most plans have "effective" or actual out-of-pocket maximums for inpatient hospital services. We also agree that in many cases these maximums can limit beneficiary inpatient cost sharing to levels below inpatient cost sharing under Medicare FFS. However, MA plans projected that about 16 percent of beneficiaries were enrolled in plans that projected higher cost sharing than under Medicare FFS even after accounting for "effective" or actual out-of-pocket maximums. While some of the 16 percent of plans may have bundled physician services with their inpatient estimates, we also showed that 80 plans with high out-of-pocket maximums for inpatient services could have higher cost sharing than Medicare FFS even with "effective" out-of-pocket maximums for inpatient hospital services.

CMS raised other concerns about our out-of-pocket maximum analysis, specifically stating that we overestimated the impact of the exclusion of Part B drugs from out-of-pocket maximums. It noted that Part B drugs administered in a physician's office would be included under an out-of-pocket maximum and that only a subset of plans excluded Part B drugs obtained from a pharmacy from the out-of-pocket maximum. We relied on the Plan Benefit Package for information regarding the analysis of Part B drug exclusions from out-of-pocket maximums. According to these data, there were 1.1 million beneficiaries in plans that reported such exclusions in 2007. We noted that the exclusions applied to Part B drugs obtained from a pharmacy and that the plans did not indicate the coverage for Part B drugs administered by a physician. We sought clarification from CMS for which Part B drugs were excluded from the out-of-pocket maximum and were told by a CMS official that plans excluded spending on Part B drugs from the out-of-pocket maximum if beneficiaries received them on an outpatient basis. We added this point of clarification to a footnote in the draft. Given CMS's subsequent agency comments on this issue, we clarified in the text that the exclusions applied to Part B drugs obtained from a pharmacy and do not typically apply to Part B drugs administered by a physician. However, we are concerned that the information in the Plan Benefit Package—information that beneficiaries rely on when they are seeking benefit coverage information—does not indicate whether chemotherapy drugs are included or excluded under the out-of-pocket maximums.

CMS also provided technical comments and clarifications, which we incorporated as appropriate.

AHIP Comment

AHIP representatives stated that they agreed with our methodology, but raised certain points that they thought the report should have made or emphasized.

AHIP representatives said that while they understood why we made a distinction between additional benefits and cost-sharing reductions, they believed that we characterized additional benefits as being the more valuable of the two. We disagreed with AHIP's assessment. While we did include a discussion of how MA plans projected they would allocate their rebates to additional benefits, premium reductions, and cost-sharing reductions, it was beyond the scope of our work to assess the relative value of the allocation options.

With regard to our cost-sharing finding, AHIP stated that while MA beneficiaries may have higher cost sharing for some categories of services, these may be offset by lower cost sharing for other categories of services. Like CMS, AHIP contended that our example of an MA plan with higher cost sharing for inpatient services, relative to FFS, did not account for the additional cost sharing Medicare FFS beneficiaries would pay for physician services during their inpatient stays. As both CMS and AHIP pointed out, most MA plans do not charge extra for physician services during inpatient stays. We have made changes to the text of our report and the accompanying figure to clarify this point. However, as our report noted, beneficiaries who frequently use high cost-sharing services could have overall cost sharing that would be higher than under Medicare FFS.

AHIP stated that although some beneficiaries may face higher cost sharing under an MA plan than if they were enrolled in Medicare FFS, their out-of-pocket costs could be lower if their MA plan has a lower premium than Medicare FFS. While this may be true in some cases—we found that, on average, plans used 3 percent of their rebates to reduce Part B premiums—it was beyond the scope of our work to make such a determination. AHIP further stated that MA plans provide beneficiaries with options. Beneficiaries who prefer more predictable expenses can choose MA plans with higher premiums and lower cost sharing, while beneficiaries who are less averse to risk can choose MA plans with lower premiums and higher cost sharing. We agree that the MA program provides beneficiaries with options and have added this point to the text of our report.

With regard to our reporting on MA plan medical loss ratios, AHIP representatives indicated that our point was fairly stated, but they asked us to mention this point in the Results in Brief section of the report. We believed that we made this point clear in our discussion of medical loss ratios and that the issue did not warrant mentioning in our high-level summary.

As agreed with your offices, unless you publicly announce the contents of this report earlier, we plan no further distribution until 30 days from its date. At that time we will send copies to the Administrator of CMS and interested congressional committees. We will also make copies available to others upon request. The report will also be available at no charge on the GAO Web site at http://www.gao.gov .

If you or your staffs have any questions about this report please contact me at (202) 512-7114 or cosgrovej@gao.gov . Contact points for our Offices of Congressional Relations and Public Affairs may be found on the last page of this report. GAO staff who made major contributions to this report are listed in appendix VI.

James C. Cosgrove
Acting Director, Health Care

List of Requesters

The Honorable John D. Dingell
Chairman
Committee on Energy and Commerce
House of Representatives

The Honorable Frank Pallone,
Jr. Chairman Subcommittee on
Health Committee on Energy and Commerce
House of Representatives

The Honorable Henry A. Waxman
Chairman
Committee on Oversight and Government Reform
House of Representatives

The Honorable Charles B. Rangel
Chairman
Committee on Ways and Means
House of Representatives

The Honorable Pete Stark
Chairman
Subcommittee on Health Committee on Ways and Means
House of Representatives

APPENDIX I. EXAMPLE OF A REBATE CALCULATION

For most Medicare Advantage (MA) plan types, Medicare provides plans with a rebate if the plan's bid is below the benchmark, but provides no rebate if the plan's bid exceeds the benchmark.[32] Table 6 is an example of rebate calculations for two hypothetical plans, both in the same county.

Both plans have the same benchmark because they are in the same county. Plan A submits a bid of $700 per member per month (PMPM). Because the plan's bid is $100 PMPM below the benchmark, it receives a rebate equal to 75 percent of that amount, or $75 PMPM. Plan A must use the $75 PMPM rebate to provide additional benefits, reduced premiums, reduced cost sharing, or any combination of the three. Plan B, however, submits a bid that is $40 PMPM above the benchmark. As a result, the plan receives no rebate. Medicare's payments to plans cannot exceed the benchmark, so Medicare's payment to Plan B is set at $800 PMPM, the amount of the benchmark. Plan B must make up the remainder of the bid by charging its beneficiaries a mandatory plan premium of $40 PMPM. Since Plan A has extra benefits and no additional premium, while Plan B has no extra benefits and an additional premium, Plan A may attract more beneficiaries. If most beneficiaries choose Plan A over Plan B, Plan B is given an incentive to become more efficient in the following year and lower its bid.

Table 6. The Calculation of the Rebate for Two Hypothetical MA Plans

	Plan A dollars per member per month	Plan B dollars per member per month
County's fee-for-service spending	$720	$720
County's benchmark	800	800
Plan bid	700	840
Amount by which bid is lower than benchmark	100	0
Plan's rebate (75 percent of amount by which bid is lower than benchmark)	75	0
Medicare payment	775	800
Mandatory plan premium	0	40
Additional benefits, reduced premiums, and		
reduced cost sharing to beneficiary	75	0

Source: GAO.

Note: All numbers in this example are standardized to represent a beneficiary of average health status.

APPENDIX II: SCOPE AND METHODOLOGY

This section describes the scope and methodology used to analyze our four objectives: (1) how MA plans projected they would allocate the rebates they receive, (2) what additional benefits MA plans commonly covered with the rebates and additional premiums, and the projected costs of these additional benefits, (3) how MA plans' projected beneficiary cost sharing, overall and by type of service, compared to Medicare fee-for-service (FFS), and (4) how MA plans projected they would allocate their revenue to medical and other expenses.

We used two primary data sources to analyze our four objectives: the 2007 Bid Pricing Tool data and the 2007 Plan Benefit Package data. These data are submitted by MA plans to the Centers for Medicare & Medicaid Services (CMS), the agency that administers Medicare. The bid pricing data contain MA plans' projections of their revenue requirements and revenue sources. Specifically, the bid pricing data include MA plans' projections of revenue requirements—spending on medical expenses, spending on non-medical expenses, and the margin. The bid pricing data also contain information on the benefits and cost-sharing arrangements of plans, including how MA plans' projected cost sharing compares to cost sharing in Medicare FFS. In addition, the bid pricing data contain information on the amount of rebates and additional premiums plans project they will require to fund additional benefits, reduced premiums, and reduced cost sharing. The benefit package data contain detailed information about the benefits and cost-sharing requirements that MA plans offer to Medicare beneficiaries.

For our objectives, we focused our analysis on plan types that account for 98 percent of MA enrollment: Health Maintenance Organizations (HMO) (71 percent), Private Fee-for-Service (PFFS) Plans (21 percent), Preferred Provider Organizations (PPO) (5 percent), and Provider-Sponsored Organizations (PSO) (1 percent).[33] We excluded Medical Savings Account plans and regional PPOs from our analysis because they follow a different bidding process. We excluded plan types that have unique restrictions on enrollment—such as employer plans, Special Needs Plans (SNP), and demonstration plans—and bids for plans that only cover Part B services. We also excluded plans with service areas that are exclusively outside the 50 states and the District of Columbia. Plans sponsors are permitted to submit separate bids for a single package of benefits by dividing the service area into segments; in these cases, benefits would be the same for each segment, but each segment's cost sharing and premiums may differ. We counted each segment as a separate plan. We used August 2007 enrollment numbers to weight our results. As a result of our methodology, we included 2,055 plans and 5,764,368 beneficiaries (71 percent of total MA enrollment) in our analysis—these numbers apply to all tables and figures in the report, unless otherwise noted. Because there were only 22 PSOs after the exclusions, and enrollment in those plans was 1 percent of MA enrollment, we do not report results separately for PSOs, but we include them in the aggregated results we report for all MA plans.

To determine how plans projected they would allocate the rebate to additional benefits, reduced premiums, and reduced cost sharing, we used the bid pricing data. The bid pricing data contain the total amounts plans projected they would spend on additional benefits, reduced premiums, and reduced cost sharing. However, since MA plans use both rebates and additional premiums as a funding source for these additional benefits, reduced premiums, and reduced cost sharing, we calculated the proportion of total funding plans projected they would spend on additional benefits, reduced premiums, and reduced cost sharing and applied these projections to the projected rebate. We restricted our analysis of rebate allocations to the 1,874 plans that received a rebate.

To identify the additional benefits that MA plans commonly covered with rebates and additional premiums, we used the benefit package data. The benefit package data provide the most detailed and accurate information about benefits offered, including additional benefits. We used the crosswalk CMS recommended—but did not require—plans to use to match service categories in the benefit package data to categories in the bid pricing data, and identified the percentage of beneficiaries in plans that offered additional benefits using bid pricing categories.[34]

To identify the costs associated with these additional benefits, we used the bid pricing data. Plans did not use consistent categories for their additional benefits in the bid pricing data. For example, some plans categorized additional vision benefits under the category of other non-covered services. Therefore, our estimates of the costs of additional benefits do not include all plans that offer those benefits, but are based on a smaller number of plans that specified that additional benefit and the associated cost of providing that benefit. In addition, some categories, such as professional services and other non-covered services, were identified by CMS as unreliable because they likely included a variety of services, and we excluded these categories from our analysis. Other categories of additional services may include some inconsistent services, and the cost estimates for additional benefits should therefore be considered as approximations.

To calculate estimated costs for each of the additional service categories, we identified plans that offered the additional benefit and that had projected a cost of at least $0.01 PMPM. The projected amounts of plans' additional benefits were adjusted for the health status of the plans' projected population by dividing the amount of the plans' additional benefits by the plans' projected risk scores—a number representing how a plan's beneficiaries' health expenditures are predicted to differ from the average beneficiary in Medicare FFS.[35] We then calculated the average amount of the additional benefit, weighting the average by the number of enrollees in the plans. If we had estimated the amount of additional benefits funded only by the rebates, the PMPM amounts of additional benefits would be lower.

To compare projected beneficiary cost sharing in MA plans and Medicare FFS, we analyzed plans' cost sharing for Medicare-covered services as reported in the bid pricing data and the equivalent Medicare FFS cost-sharing amounts, also included in the bid pricing data. The equivalent Medicare FFS cost sharing represents an MA beneficiary's expected cost sharing under Medicare FFS if the beneficiary's MA plan had the same pricing and utilization as Medicare FFS. The Medicare FFS equivalent cost sharing for each service category was calculated by applying the average cost-sharing percentage under Medicare FFS for a given service category to each plan's total cost estimates for providing benefits in that service category. For example, if the cost-sharing percentage under Medicare FFS for inpatient services is 10 percent for a given county, and an MA plan in that county projects spending on inpatient services at $200 PMPM, then the equivalent inpatient cost sharing is 10 percent of $200, or $20 PMPM. For Part A services, the cost-sharing percentage under Medicare FFS is calculated for each county—one county may have an equivalent inpatient cost-sharing percentage of 10 percent, while another county may have a percentage of 8 percent. For Part B services, however, the cost-sharing percentages are a national average, so the same percentages were applied to all counties. We divided each plan's estimated cost sharing and the Medicare equivalent cost sharing by each plan's projected risk score to get estimated cost sharing for a beneficiary with average Medicare health spending. We reported the percentage of plans that had cost sharing higher than the estimated Medicare cost sharing for a given service category.

When we calculated the amount of reduced cost sharing, we used the total amounts reported in the bid pricing data. We included both rebates and additional premiums because this provided the accurate amount of cost-sharing reductions that MA plans projected their beneficiaries will receive. The amounts of the additional benefits and cost-sharing reductions in our analyses would be lower if we had restricted our analysis to rebates as the sole funding source.

To determine plans' out-of-pocket maximums, we examined the in-network out-of-pocket maximum and the combined out-of-pocket maximum (a maximum that applies to both in-network and out-of-network services) fields in the benefit package data. If the two fields were the same value, then we defined the out-of-pocket maximum as equal to that value. If one of the fields was blank, and the other field was a positive number, then we defined the out-of-pocket maximum as equal to the value of the field with the positive number. If both fields had a positive number, but they were not equal, then we defined the out-of-pocket maximum as equal to the value of the field with the lower value. We categorized a plan as having an out-of-pocket maximum even if the plan excluded certain categories of service from that maximum. We did not categorize a plan that had only a service-specific maximum as having an out-of-pocket maximum.

To determine the percentage of total revenue allocated to medical expenses and other expenses, we used the bid pricing data and calculated the projected values of medical expenses, non-medical expenses, and margin as a percentage of revenue for all plans and by plan type.[36] We reported the percentages of beneficiaries in plans that projected medical expenses less than 85 percent. We also analyzed the percentage of revenue projected to go to sales and marketing from the bid pricing data.

APPENDIX III: PLAN VARIATION IN REBATE AMOUNTS

Rebate amounts, as well as the allocation of rebates, varied considerably from plan to plan. To provide a measure of this variation, we calculated rebate amounts and the amounts of additional benefits, reduced premiums, and reduced cost sharing at the 25th and 75th percentiles, weighted for enrollment. A percentile is

Table 7. Rebate Amount Allocated to Additional Benefits, Premium Reductions, and Cost-Sharing Reductions by Plan Type, 2007

Average	HMO Plans = 1,179 Beneficiaries = 3,747,087	PFFS Plans = 367 Beneficiaries = 1,361,668	PPO Plans = 306 Beneficiaries = 268,460	All plans[a] Plans = 1,874 Beneficiaries = 5,454,573
Rebate total				
25th percentile	$57.81	$59.70	$37.33	$56.32
75th percentile	118.19	83.30	69.83	108.55
Amount of rebate allocated to Additional benefits[b]				
25th percentile	4.14	0.00	3.56	2.75
75th percentile	15.51	11.41	13.96	13.70
Part D premium reduction[c]				
25th percentile	0.21	0.00	0.00	0.00
75th percentile	24.04	24.12	7.25	24.12
Part B premium reduction				
25th percentile	0.00	0.00	0.00	0.00
75th percentile	0.00	0.00	0.00	0.00
Cost-sharing reduction[b]				
25th percentile	42.89	39.02	26.79	39.02
75th percentile	84.88	68.95	52.60	78.90

Source: GAO analysis of 2007 CMS Bid Pricing Tool data.

Notes: Values are weighted by August 2007 plan enrollment and are standardized to represent a beneficiary of average health status. Employer plans, Part B only plans, SNPs, regional PPOs, and plans with service areas that are exclusively outside of the 50 states and the District of Columbia were excluded from the analysis. There were 1,874 plans that received a rebate.

[a] The "All plans" category includes HMOs, PFFS plans, PPOs, and PSOs. Results are not reported separately for PSOs because there were only 22 PSO plans and enrollment in those plans constituted1 percent of total MA enrollment.

[b] The rebate amounts allocated toward cost sharing and additional benefits included some non-medical expenses, such as administrative costs and plans' margins.

[c] Of 1,874 plans that received a rebate, 1,423 offered Part D benefits to their beneficiaries. Of those that offered Part D, 1,037 reduced Part D premiums.

the value below which a certain percentage of beneficiaries fall. For example, the value of the cost-sharing reduction at the 25th percentile was $39.02 PMPM and at the 75th percentile was $78.90 PMPM, meaning that at least 25 percent of beneficiaries were in plans that projected a cost-sharing reduction of $39.02 PMPM or less, and at least 75 percent of beneficiaries were in plans that projected a cost-sharing reduction of $78.90 PMPM or less. (See table 7.)

APPENDIX IV: PLAN VARIATION IN THE OUT-OF-POCKET MAXIMUM

In 2007, about half of MA beneficiaries were in plans that had an out-of-pocket maximum, a dollar limit on a beneficiary's cost sharing. The out-of-pocket maximum varied from plan to plan. To provide a measure of this out-of-pocket maximum variation, we calculated the out-of-pocket maximum at the 25th and 75th percentiles, weighted for enrollment. A percentile is the value below which a certain percentage of beneficiaries fall. For example, the out-of-pocket maximum at the 25th percentile was $2,750, and at the 75th percentile it was $4,600,

Table 8. Variation in Values of Out-of-Pocket Maximum by Plan Type,

	Plan type			
	HMO Plans = 444 Beneficiaries = 1,436,148	**PFFS** Plans = 350 Beneficiaries = 1,087,383	**PPO** Plans = 219 Beneficiaries = 205,713	**All plans[a]** Plans = 1,016 Beneficiaries = 2,738,531
Value of out-of-pocket maximum				
Average	$3,204	$4,026	$2,377	$3,463
25th percentile	2,750	3,000	1,000	2,750
75th percentile	4,000	5,000	3,100	4,600

Source: GAO analysis of 2007 CMS Plan Benefit Package data.

Notes: Values are weighted by plan enrollment. If a plan had two out-of-pocket maximums—one for in-network services and one for combined in- and out-of-network services, then we used the lower value for this analysis. Determination of a plan's overall out-of-pocket maximum did not take into account whether a plan had a maximum for a specific category of service. Employer plans, Part B only plans, SNPs, regional PPOs, and plans with service areas that are exclusively outside of the 50 states and the District of Columbia were excluded from the analysis.

[a] The "All plans" category includes HMOs, PFFS plans, PPOs, and PSOs. Results are not reported separately for PSOs because there were only 22 PSO plans and enrollment in those plans constituted 1 percent of total MA enrollment.

meaning that at least 25 percent of beneficiaries were in plans with an out-of-pocket maximum $2,750 or less, and at least 75 percent of beneficiaries were in plans with an out-of-pocket maximum of $4,600 or less. (See table 8.)

APPENDIX V: COMMENTS FROM THE CENTERS FOR MEDICARE & MEDICAID SERVICES

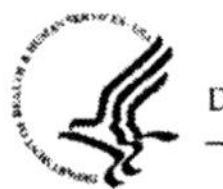

DEPARTMENT OF HEALTH & HUMAN SERVICES

Centers for Medicare & Medicaid Services

Office of the Administrator
Washington, DC 20201

FEB - 1 2008

DATE:

TO: James C. Cosgrove
Director, Health Care
Government Accountability Office

FROM: Kerry Weems
Acting Administrator

SUBJECT: Government Accountability Office (GAO) Draft Report: MEDICARE ADVANTAGE: Increased Spending Relative to Medicare Fee for Service May Not Always Reduce Beneficiary Out of Pocket Costs (GAO-08-359)

Thank you for the opportunity to review and comment on the GAO draft report referenced above. In this draft report, the GAO examined (1) Medicare Advantage (MA) plans' projected rebate reallocations; (2) additional benefits MA plans commonly covered and their costs; (3) MA plans' projected cost-sharing; and (4) MA plans' allocation of projected revenues and expenses.

General Comments

Inpatient Cost Sharing:

The report finds that out of pocket costs for inpatient services are more than double for 16 percent of MA enrollees than in Fee-For-Service (FFS). We do not disagree with the findings; however the report does not address a number of areas that mitigate the impact of the finding:

(1) MA bundling of cost sharing versus unbundled FFS cost sharing: We believe that GAO did not take into consideration that an inpatient stay under FFS is not comprised of just the deductible amount for each hospitalization. It also contains a professional service charge which is billed to the beneficiary. As an example of the type of expense incurred by a FFS beneficiary for a 90-day hospital stay, the average professional service co-pay under FFS alone is equal to $5,286. MA enrollees do not receive a separate bill for professional services. The cost of these Part B services were not incorporated into the GAO analysis and therefore overstate the effect of inpatient cost sharing on the possible MA enrollees cited in the draft report.

2) MA is more protective for longer hospitalizations than FFS: The report also does not contemplate the FFS costs for a long hospitalization (e.g., more than 15 days) compared to a long hospitalization under MA. The Centers for Medicare & Medicaid Services (CMS) has data to show that MA plans have lower cost sharing for an inpatient stay than an FFS stay for longer stays – for example 95 percent of MA plans have a lower cost share than FFS for a 90-day stay.

Page 2 - James C. Cosgrove

and 85 percent of MA plans have a lower cost share than FFS for a 25-day stay. Figure 4 on Page 21 is misleading in that it only compares out-of-pocket costs for 15 days of hospitalization or less. Less healthy beneficiaries may have longer than 15-day hospitalizations in a year. We would recommend providing longer inpatient hospitalization information and a figure demonstrating it to give a more balanced perspective on inpatient hospitalizations.

3) The report does not address effective out-of-pocket maxes for inpatient stays: Maximum out-of-pocket values in the plan benefit package (PBP) data are not the only way to specify the maximum amount an enrollee will pay for a specific benefit. For example, a plan showing no out of pocket maximum value in its PBP but having a $200 per day copay for days 1 through 6 of inpatient stays has an *effective* maximum enrollee out-of-pocket cost of $1,200 for inpatient stays regardless of the length of stay. In fact, most plans "max out" their out of pocket costs for inpatient stays at values far less than those for FFS. Our data show that, for the same population of plans GAO includes, 74 percent of enrollees in 2007 were in plans having an effective maximum out of pocket for inpatient stays of $1,000 or less and nearly 100 percent of enrollees were in plans having an effective maximum out of pocket costs less than the FFS Medicare value.

4) Misrepresentations of data in text, table and figures on inpatient cost sharing:

- Footnote b to Table 4 states: "In some cases, MA plans include cost sharing for professional services, such as physician visits in, in the inpatient category." We believe that because plans include professional services in the bundled inpatient cost sharing, the data in Table 4 is a misrepresentation of a true comparison between MA inpatient cost sharing and FFS inpatient cost sharing. That is, inpatient cost sharing for MA will naturally look higher than FFS in your table because of the inclusion of professional services under the inpatient services category for MA.

- Also, about 1/3 of Medicare FFS inpatient admissions fall within an existing benefit period resulting in no beneficiary liability for the Part A deductible. Also, FFS beneficiaries are required to pay cost sharing beginning on day 61 of an inpatient admission. Further, FFS beneficiaries are required to pay certain Part B cost sharing for care provided in inpatient facilities. Accordingly, the FFS representation in Figure 4 has an incorrect level and slope, and we suggest that the chart be modified accordingly, or removed from the report.

5) Part B Drugs and out-of-pocket exclusion and more than 1 million affected enrollees: We believe that the number and impact contained in the report is overstated. Part B drugs administered in a physician's office would be included under an out-of-pocket cap because the bill for the Part B coinsurance would be incurred as a physician office visit. The exclusion of Part B drugs from out of pocket maximums is for those drugs obtained from a pharmacy (as opposed to at the physician's office). We believe Part B drugs obtained at the pharmacy represents a subset of the 2007 plans with a Part B drugs out-of-pocket maximum exclusion.

Page 3 - James C. Cosgrove

6) We believe that the report misses the fact that the majority of MA benefit packages in 2007 are better and are more protective for out-of-pocket costs than FFS. Overall, MA benefit packages in 2007 are richer than FFS. Some examples include:

- MA plans are not required to cap out-of-pocket expenses for enrollees; however, almost one-half (48 percent in 2007) cap out-of-pocket expenses for enrollees, making them far more protective than an FFS beneficiary who has no cap on out-of-pocket costs.
- 72.8 percent of enrollees are in plans with a 21-day inpatient psychiatric stay cost less than that of FFS.
- 93.6 percent of enrollees are in plans with an out-of-pocket cost for annual renal visits (dialysis) less than that of FFS.
- 98.4 percent of eligibles have access to a plan with a maximum out-of-pocket value of $3,150 or less that includes key specific benefit categories.
- 87.3 percent of the plans cover additional inpatient hospital days beyond the FFS allowed 90-day maximum.

7) We believe that the report fails to acknowledge that MA plans provide beneficiaries with a variety of choices in benefit structures other than original Medicare. These choices allow beneficiaries to select a benefit structure that best suits their medical needs while taking their financial considerations into account. For example, some beneficiaries may prefer to pay lower cost-sharing for some Medicare benefits that they anticipate using during the year, and are willing to accept the risk of paying higher cost-sharing on other benefits should they need them.

8) We are also concerned that this report is unfairly skewed. To name a few that we believe should be addressed:

- The title is misleading and does not reflect the content of the report. GAO report titles should be neutral, or, at least, not misrepresent the contents of the report.
- On page 1 of the report, the discussion of the payment increases based on the Medicare Prescription Drug, Improvement and Modernization Act of 2003 fails to address the intention of Congress to expand access to MA plans in rural areas.
- The presentation of MA plans that offer cost sharing that is higher than Medicare FFS does not provide a similarly structured presentation of examples of plans offering cost sharing lower than FFS. As such, the report relies on outlier plan designs (high inpatient cost sharing) with outlier plan services (e.g. long inpatient lengths of stay) to make its point.

End Notes

[1] Medicare is the federally financed health insurance program for persons aged 65 and over, certain individuals with disabilities, and individuals with end-stage renal disease. Medicare Part A covers hospital and other inpatient stays. Medicare Part B is optional insurance, and covers hospital outpatient, physician, and other services. Medicare Parts A and B are known as original Medicare or Medicare FFS. Medicare beneficiaries have the option of obtaining coverage for Medicare Part A and B services from private health plans that participate in Medicare's MA program—also known as Medicare Part C. All Medicare beneficiaries may purchase coverage for outpatient prescription drugs under Medicare Part D.

[2] Pub. L. No. 108-173, § 201, et. seq., 117 Stat. 2066, 2176.

[3] Private health plans had previously provided heath coverage to Medicare beneficiaries through the Medicare + Choice program. MMA renamed the program "Medicare Advantage" and changed certain payments and other aspects of the program.

[4] Medicare Payment Advisory Commission' *The Medicare Advantage Program and MedPAC Recommendations* (Washington, D.C.: April 2007).

[5] Congressional Budget Office, *The Medicare Advantage Program: Enrollment Trends and Budgetary Effects* (Washington, D.C.: April 2007).

[6] For a discussion of Medicare's long-term financial challenges, see GAO, *Long-Term Budget Outlook: Saving Our Future Requires Tough Choices Today*, GAO-07-342T (Washington, D.C.: Jan. 11, 2007).

[7] Medicare compares a plan's bid to the benchmark after adjusting the benchmark to reflect the health status of the plan's enrollees.

[8] About 95 percent of MA beneficiaries are in plans that receive rebates and 41 percent of MA beneficiaries are in plans that charge additional premiums. Some plans also offer optional benefits, which beneficiaries can purchase with the standard benefit package. Rebates can not be used for optional benefits.

[9] Margins, sometimes referred to as profits, refer to plans' remaining revenue after medical and non-medical expenses are paid. In certain circumstances, such as for new market entrants, CMS allows a plan to have a negative margin, meaning that the plan's revenue is less than its combined medical and non-medical expenses.

[10] HMOs account for 71 percent of total MA enrollment; PFFS plans 21 percent; PPOs 5 percent; and PSOs 1 percent, totaling to 98 percent of enrollment. The remaining 2 percent of beneficiaries were enrolled in Medical Savings Accounts and regional PPOs. Beneficiaries in HMOs are generally restricted to seeing providers within a network, while PFFS beneficiaries can see any provider that accepts the plan's payment terms. Beneficiaries in PPOs can see both in-network and out-of-network providers but must pay higher cost-sharing amounts if they use out-of-network services. PSOs are MA plans that are operated by a provider or providers.

[11] Some MA plans only cover Medicare Part B services.

[12] MA plans do not cover hospice care, a benefit that is provided under Medicare FFS.

[13] U.S. citizens and permanent residents meet Medicare's work requirement if they worked for at least 10 years in Medicare-covered employment or if their spouse worked for at least 10 years in Medicare-covered employment.

[14] Beneficiaries who are also eligible for Medicaid can have their Part B premium paid for by their state Medicaid program.

[15] Individuals with end-stage renal disease are not eligible for most MA plans, unless they develop the disease while enrolled in an MA plan. 42 U.S.C. § 1395w-21(a)(3)(B)(2000).

[16] Many Medicare FFS beneficiaries pay premiums for a type of supplemental insurance known as Medigap, which limits beneficiary cost sharing for Medicare-covered services. Medigap policies do not cover the cost sharing of MA beneficiaries.

[17] CMS officials said that the thresholds that trigger further review by CMS are at or above Medicare FFS cost-sharing levels. For example, in 2007 Medicare FFS beneficiaries were charged a $992 deductible for hospital services, so the cost-sharing threshold was at or above $992.

[18] CMS officials indicated that in evaluating 2008 plans, they stratified plans based on having an out-of-pocket maximum of $3,250, instead of $3,100.

[19] The rebate amounts allocated to cost sharing include some non-medical expenses, such as administrative costs and plans' margins.

[20] The average additional premium has been standardized to represent a beneficiary of average health status.

[21] The 888 plans that received a rebate and did not charge an additional premium projected that they would allocate 11 percent ($11 PMPM) of their rebate to additional benefits, 21 percent ($22 PMPM) to Part D premium reductions, 3 percent ($4 PMPM) to Part B premium reductions, and 65 percent ($70 PMPM) to cost-sharing reductions. The 986 plans that charged additional premiums and received a rebate projected that they would allocate 14 percent ($8 PMPM) of their rebate to additional benefits, 3 percent ($2 PMPM) to Part D premium reductions, 0 percent ($0 PMPM) to Part B premium reductions, and 83 percent ($44 PMPM) to cost-sharing reductions. These numbers are enrollment weighted.

[22] Some categories were identified by CMS as unreliable and were excluded from our analysis.

[23] Average cost sharing reflects expenditures for the entire population and includes both beneficiaries who are projected to use a certain category of service and beneficiaries who are not projected to use that service.

[24] Medicare FFS beneficiaries could have paid the deductible more than once for multiple visits under some circumstances. The 2007 deductible was $992 for each benefit period. Under Medicare FFS, a benefit period begins the day a beneficiary enters a hospital, skilled nursing facility, or critical access hospital, and it ends when the beneficiary has not been an inpatient of a hospital, skilled nursing facility, or critical access hospital for 60 consecutive days. A Medicare FFS beneficiary who had three hospital stays in one benefit period in 2007 would have paid a $992 deductible, while a beneficiary who had three hospital stays in three separate benefit periods would have paid a $992 deductible for each hospital stay, or $2,976.

[25] The plans either had no out-of-pocket maximum or had a maximum that was above $3,100. In addition, the plans had no service-specific maximum for inpatient services.

[26] The average length of stay in Medicare FFS was 5.4 days in 2005, according to a MedPAC analysis of Medicare cost report data. For plans with no out-of-pocket maximum and a per day copayment of $200 or more for the first 10 hospital days, beneficiaries would have been billed at least $2,000 for a 10-day hospital stay and at least $3,000 for three stays that are each 5 days long. However, beneficiaries in plans with an out-of-pocket maximum and a per day copayment of $200 or more could have been billed less than these amounts if they had already paid cost sharing for other categories of services. About 15 percent of hospital stays under Medicare lasted 10 days or more in 2004, according to CMS data.

[27] Medicare FFS does not have an out-of-pocket maximum. However, Medicare FFS beneficiaries who have supplemental insurance can have some or all of their cost sharing paid for. Medicare FFS beneficiaries who buy Medigap insurance have their Part A and Part B cost sharing paid for by their Medigap plan, although they still may pay deductibles. Medicare FFS beneficiaries with Medicaid and with employer plans can also have some or all of their cost sharing paid for by their plan. As of 2004, 26 percent of Medicare beneficiaries had Medigap insurance, 17 percent had Medicaid, and 38 percent had employer insurance, with some beneficiaries having more than one type of supplemental insurance. Data are based on MedPAC's analysis of the 2004 Medicare Current Beneficiary Survey.

[28] A plan was considered to have excluded a service category from the out-of-pocket maximum if the out-of-pocket maximum did not cover that service category and if the plan had no service-specific maximum for that category.

[29] Non-medical expenses include administration, marketing, and sales. Margin is the amount of revenue above or below the revenue needed to cover medical and non-medical expenses.

Allocations to medical expenses, non-medical expenses, and margins do not add to $783 PMPM due to rounding.

30 There is no definitive standard for what a medical loss ratio should be. For example, the CHAMP Act, H.R. 3162, 110th Cong., § 414 (2007), which was passed in the House of Representatives on August 1, 2007, included a medical loss ratio threshold of 0.85. In contrast, individual Medigap policies are currently required to achieve a medical loss ratio of at least 0.65, while group Medigap policies are required to achieve a medical loss ratio of at least 0.75. AHIP reported that from 1960 to 2003, the medical loss ratio for private plans averaged about 0.88.

31 Direct administration accounts for functions that are directly related to the administration of the MA program, such as customer service and medical management. Indirect administration accounts for functions that may be considered "corporate services," such as accounting operations and human resources. Private reinsurance is the insurance provided by another company that assumes financial risk previously assumed by the MA plan. The net cost of private reinsurance is equal to the reinsurance premium less projected reinsurance recoveries.

32 For Medical Savings Account (MSA) plans, Medicare makes a deposit into a beneficiary's savings account if the bid is lower than the benchmark, instead of providing the plan with a rebate. Regional Preferred Provider Organizations (PPO) can receive rebates, but their benchmarks are determined differently than local plans. Due to these differences, the example in this appendix does not refer to MSA plans and regional PPOs.

33 Percentage of MA enrollment by plan type is based on August 2007 enrollment.

34 Centers for Medicare & Medicaid Services, *Instructions for Completing the Medicare Advantage Bid Pricing Tool For Contract Year 2007* (Baltimore, Md.: May 2006).

35 If a plan has a population with health expenditures that on average are the same as those for Medicare FFS, then the plan would have a risk score of one. If a plan has a population with projected health expenditures that on average are greater than or less than those for an average beneficiary in Medicare FFS, then the plan's risk score would be greater than or less than one, respectively.

36 The bid pricing data exclude the additional revenue requirements for beneficiaries with end-stage renal disease from this calculation.

In: Medicare Advantage: The Alternate Medicare … ISBN: 978-1-60876-031-2
Editors: Charles V. Baylis, pp.133-147

Chapter 4

MEDICARE ADVANTAGE ORGANIZATIONS: ACTUAL EXPENSES AND PROFITS COMPARED TO PROJECTIONS FOR 2006

United States Government Accountability Office

December 8, 2008

The Honorable Pete Stark
Chairman
Subcommittee on Health
Committee on Ways and Means
House of Representatives

Subject: *Medicare Advantage Organizations: Actual Expenses and Profits Compared to Projections for 2006*

Dear Mr. Chairman:

The federal government's spending on the Medicare Advantage (MA) program has grown substantially in recent years, from approximately $60 billion in 2006 and $77 billion in 2007 to an estimated $91 billion in 2008.[1] MA organizations provide health care coverage to Medicare beneficiaries through private health plans, thus offering an alternative to the original Medicare fee-for-service (FFS) program.[2] Payments to MA organizations are, in part, based on the projected expenditures organizations submit in their bids for providing Medicare-covered services, as well as actual enrollment and beneficiary health status. Once Medicare payments are determined, they are not modified based on differences between actual and projected expenses.[3] MA organizations are not required to submit claims data to the Centers for Medicare & Medicaid Services (CMS)—the agency that administers Medicare—but they must report actual expenditures for the year 2 years prior to the upcoming contract year. For example, MA organizations reported their actual 2006 expenditures in their bid submission for contract year 2008. When MA organizations submit their bids, the actual expenditures reported in their bid submissions reflect the MA organizations' most recent full calendar year of actual expenditure data.

In June 2008, we reported that for 2005, MA organizations generally spent less on medical expenses and earned more profits than projected.[4] MA organizations' self-reported actual profit margin was approximately 5 percent of total revenue, on average, which was approximately $1.1 billion more in 2005 than MA organizations had projected.

The accuracy of MA organizations' projections is important because, in addition to determining Medicare payments, these projections also affect the extent to which MA beneficiaries receive additional benefits not provided under FFS and the amounts beneficiaries pay in cost sharing and premiums. For example, if MA organizations had more accurately projected their revenues and expenses in 2005, they would have been able to provide beneficiaries with additional benefits or cost-sharing reductions, and still maintain the level of profits projected.

This report responds to your request for updated information on the accuracy of MA organizations' projections. Specifically, this report compares MA organizations' 2006 actual medical expenses, non-medical expenses, and profits to projections for the same year, and compares 2006 results to 2005 results. When we requested data from CMS, 2006 was the most recent year for which data were available.

To report MA organizations' actual expenditures, actual profits and projections for 2006, we analyzed the two-year look-back form that MA organizations submitted in 2007 to CMS with the 2008 Bid Pricing Tool.[5] The 2008 two-year look-back form contains MA organizations' selfreported actual medical expenses, non-medical expenses, and profits for 2006, in addition to the projections for 2006 the organizations submitted in 2005.[6] MA organizations submit a single two-year look-back form for each of their contracts, which may include more than one health benefit plan. We excluded employer group health plans because these plans are not open to the general Medicare population, and actual and projected expenses are calculated differently than for other plans. We also excluded small contracts, defined as those with fewer than 24,000 "member months" (equivalent to 2,000 beneficiaries enrolled for a full year), because CMS officials stated they do not consider data from these contracts to be fully credible.[7] Additionally, we excluded two contracts for which actual or projected expenditures were missing. After all exclusions, our analysis included 224 contracts, representing about 57 percent of the contracts for which a two-year look-back form was submitted and about 84 percent of MA enrollment, equivalent to approximately 5.6 million beneficiaries enrolled in contracted plans for a full year. Within our sample of contracts, we analyzed data for three different plan types: Health Maintenance Organizations (HMO), Private Fee-for-Service (PFFS) plans, and Preferred Provider Organizations (PPO).[8] These plan types account for 82 percent of enrollment and 55 percent of contracts for which a two-year look-back form was submitted. To determine actual and projected expenses and profits for 2005 and 2006, we multiplied both actual and projected per member per month expenses and profits by actual enrollment in member months for that year. To compute average actual and projected expenses and profits as a percentage of revenue, we weighted each MA organization's percentage by its total revenue. This approach differs slightly from the enrollment weighting approach we used in our June 2008 report, although the two approaches yield nearly identical results. The percentages reported in our June 2008 report are included in the background section. Results are reported for the specific contract year and may not be representative of or generalizable to other contract years.

We interviewed officials at CMS about data reliability and reviewed all data for reasonableness and consistency; while we did not independently audit MA organizations' selfreported data, we were able to determine that the data were sufficiently reliable for our purposes. We conducted this performance audit from October 2008 to November 2008, in accordance with generally accepted government auditing standards. Those standards require that we plan and perform the audit to obtain sufficient, appropriate evidence to provide a reasonable basis for our findings and conclusions based on our audit objectives. We believe that the evidence obtained provides a reasonable basis for our findings and conclusions based on our audit objectives.

RESULTS IN BRIEF

On average, MA organizations reported earning profits of 6.6 percent of total revenue in 2006—which was higher than their projected profits of 4.1 percent. MA organizations reported spending an average of 83.3 percent of total revenue on medical expenses, but had projected spending an average of 86.9 percent of total revenue on those expenses. More than half of beneficiaries were enrolled in health benefits plans offered by MA organizations for which profits as a percentage of revenue were greater than projected and the combined medical and non-medical expenses as a percentage of revenue were lower than projected. Among the three types of MA health plans with the largest enrollments—HMOs, PPOs, and PFFS plans—there was a consistent pattern of actual profits being higher than projected and medical expenses being lower than projected. Projections of profits were closer to actual profits as a percentage of revenue in 2006 (2.5 percentage points difference) than they were in 2005 (3.2 percentage points difference). However, largely due to an approximate 40 percent increase in enrollment between the 2 years, the actual dollar amount of the difference between actual and projected profits increased from $1.1 billion in 2005 to $1.3 billion in 2006.

In commenting on a draft of our report, CMS stated that it agreed with our findings. In addition, CMS stated that the small difference between MA organizations' actual and projected aggregate medical expenses was within the prevailing range of such differences for a 1-year-ahead estimate. CMS further noted that MA organizations' higher-than-projected profits were due primarily to higher-than-projected revenues from Medicare. As we stated in our report, however, if MA organizations had more accurately projected both their revenues and expenses, they would have been able to provide beneficiaries with additional benefits or cost-sharing reductions, and still maintain the level of profits projected.

BACKGROUND

Organizations that participate in Medicare's program for private health plans have been required to submit projections of their expenses and profits to CMS since the 1980s.[9] Beginning in 2006, MA organizations have been required to submit bids to CMS that reflect their projected revenue requirements for the medical expenses, non-medical expenses, and profit margin associated with offering the same benefits available in the FFS program.[10] Medicare pays an MA organization an amount per member per month based on the relationship between the organization's bid and an administratively set rate known as a benchmark. Benchmarks are the maximum amount Medicare will pay an organization to serve an average beneficiary, and while they vary by county, every county in the United States had a benchmark that was at least as high as the average spending per member per month for all FFS Medicare enrollees in that county. If an MA organization's bid is higher than the benchmark, Medicare pays the organization the amount of the benchmark, and the organization must charge beneficiaries a premium to collect the amount by which the bid exceeds the benchmark. If an MA organization's bid is lower than the benchmark, the organization receives the amount of the bid plus additional payments, known as rebates, equal to 75 percent of the difference between the benchmark and the bid.[11] MA organizations are required to spend their rebates on additional benefits, reduced cost sharing, reduced premiums, or a combination of the three.

In June 2008, we reported that for 2005, on average, MA organizations reported that they spent less on medical expenses and earned more profits than projected.[12] MA organizations, on average, reported spending 85.7 percent of total revenue on medical expenses in 2005, but had projected medical expenditures of 90.2 percent of total revenue. On average, MA organizations' self-reported actual profit margin was 5.1 percent of total revenue compared to a projected profit margin of 1.8 percent of total revenue, which is approximately $1.1 billion more in 2005 than MA organizations had projected.[13] In commenting on a draft of that report, CMS stated that the finding was not relevant to assessment of the MA program because the payment system in 2005 was different from the current competitive bidding process, which took effect in 2006. CMS stated that the competitive bidding model brought market discipline to the Medicare program, and consisted of a rigorous system of actuarial bid submissions that were subject to careful review by the Office of the Actuary at CMS.

Profits and Non-Medical Expenses Were Higher While Medical Expenses Were Lower Than Projected, on Average

MA organizations' self-reported profits and non-medical expenses were, on average, higher in 2006 than they had projected, while medical expenses were lower than projected. Specifically, MA organizations reported, on average, earning profits of 6.6 percent of total revenue in 2006—which was higher than their projected profits of 4.1 percent. Actual nonmedical expenses (10.1 percent of total revenue) were higher than projected (9.0 percent of total revenue) as well. MA organizations reported spending an average of 83.3 percent of total revenue on medical expenses, but had projected spending an average of 86.9 percent of total revenue on those expenses.

MA organizations included in our analysis received $1.7 billion more in revenues than projected, based on the actual number of enrolled beneficiaries.[14] CMS officials stated that changes in the mix and health status of projected versus actually enrolled beneficiaries may have produced differences between actual expenditures and projections. That is, MA organizations received higher-than-projected revenues because Medicare paid additional amounts to compensate for enrollees who were deemed potentially more costly because of their health status,[15] who were disproportionately from counties with higher benchmarks, who were disproportionately enrolled in more expensive plans, or a combination of the three. The MA organizations' aggregate data show, however, that the increased payments were not accompanied by commensurately higher-than-projected expenses. MA organizations selfreported spending slightly less on medical expenses ($42.2 billion) than the amount projected ($42.5 billion), and slightly more on non-medical expenses ($5.1 billion) than the amount projected ($4.4 billion). Overall, actual expenses ($47.3 billion) were about the same as projected ($46.9 billion). Consequently, MA organizations earned $1.3 billion more in profits than projected in 2006. (See table 1.)

More than half of beneficiaries were enrolled in health benefits plans offered by MA organizations for which actual profits were greater than projections as a percentage of revenue. More than two-thirds of beneficiaries were enrolled in health benefit plans for which actual medical expenses were less than projections as a percentage of revenue. In contrast, more than two-thirds of beneficiaries were enrolled in plans for which actual non-medical expenses were greater than projections as a percentage of revenue. (See figure 1.)

Among the three types of MA health plans with the largest enrollments—HMOs, PPOs, and PFFS plans—there was a consistent pattern of actual profits being higher than projected and medical expenses being lower than projected. On average, HMO plans reported the largest profit margin as a percentage of total revenue (7.2 percent) whereas PFFS plans reported the smallest (3.1 percent). (See table 2.) PPO plans reported spending the highest percentage of total revenue on medical expenses (85.5 percent) while PFFS plans reported thc smallest (81.3 percent). PFFS plans reported spending 15.6 percent of total revenue on non-medical expenses, more than HMO plans (9.4 percent) or PPO plans (10.5 percent) and more than 50 percent greater than what they projected.

In 2006, MA organizations had greater profits as a percentage of revenue (6.6 percent) than in 2005 (5.0 percent).[16] (See table 3.) Although the increase in profits as a percentage of revenue from 2005 to 2006 was only 1.6 percentage points, MA organizations' aggregate profits nearly doubled from 2005 to 2006. The increase was largely driven by the approximate 40 percent increase in enrollment between the 2 years.

MA organizations in aggregate earned $1.3 billion more in profits than projected in 2006, compared to $1.1 billion more in profits than projected in 2005. While the difference between actual and projected profits as a percentage of revenue in 2006 (2.5 percentage points) was less than the difference in 2005 (3.2 percentage points), the total difference between actual and projected profits was greater because of enrollment growth. The median amount of actual profits earned above projections per contract was approximately $1.7 million in 2006, compared to the 2005 median of $2.8 million actual profits above projected.[17]

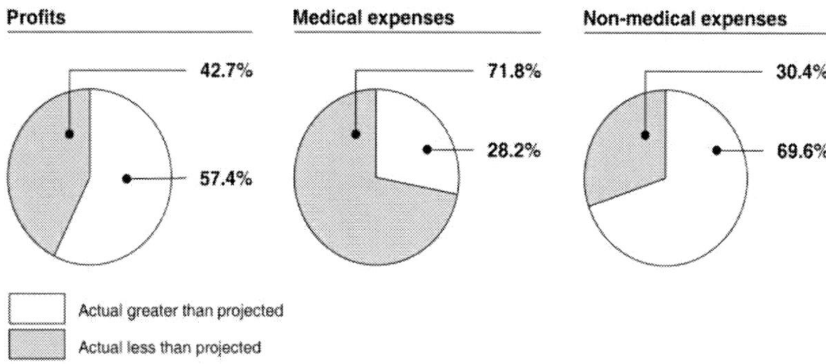

Source: CMS.

Notes: Data on actual expenses and profits were self-reported by MA organizations. Percentage totals may add to more than 100 due to rounding. We used member months as our measure of beneficiary enrollment. Twelve member months is equivalent to one beneficiary enrolled in a contracted plan for a full year. We excluded from our analysis employer group health plans and contracts for which revenue projections or actual expenditures were not reported. We also excluded from our analysis contracts that had fewer than 24,000 member months, which is equivalent to 2,000 beneficiaries enrolled for a full year. The analysis includes 224 contracts, representing about 57 percent of the contracts for which a two-year look-back form was submitted and about 84 percent of MA enrollment, equivalent to approximately 5.6 million beneficiaries enrolled in contracted plans for a full year.

Figure 1. Percentage of Beneficiaries Covered by MA Organizations with Reported Expenses and Profits as a Percentage of Revenue That Were Greater Than or Less Than Projections, 2006

Table 1. Actual and Projected Medical Expenses, Non-Medical Expenses, and Profits as Amounts and Percentages of Revenue, 2006

	Actual			Projected		
	Percentage of revenue	**Amount in dollars per beneficiary**	**Amount in dollars (billions)**	**Percentage of revenue**	**Amount in dollars per beneficiary**	**Amount in dollars (billions)**
Medical expenses[a]	83.3	7,551.38	42.15	86.9	7,614.39	42.51
Non-medical expenses	10.1	913.59	5.10	9.0	785.72	4.39
Profits	6.6	601.79	3.36	4.1	363.13	2.03
Total Revenue[b]		**9,066.76**	**50.61**		**8,763.24**	**48.92**

Source: CMS.

Notes: Data on actual expenses and profits were self-reported by MA organizations. Percentages are weighted total revenue. Percentage totals may add to less than 100 due to rounding. We excluded from our analysis employer group health plans and contracts for which revenue projections or actual expenditures were not reported. We also excluded from our analysis contracts that had fewer than 24,000 member months, which is equivalent to 2,000 beneficiaries enrolled for a full year. The analysis includes 224 contracts, representing about 57 percent of the contracts for which a two-year look-back form was submitted and about 84 percent of MA enrollment, equivalent to approximately 5.6 million beneficiaries enrolled in contracted plans for a full year.

[a] A CMS official we spoke with stated that medical expenses as a percentage of revenue may vary for reasons other than utilization and cost of providing care. Some MA organizations, for example, may categorize the costs of delivering caremanagement services as medical expenses, while other MA organizations may classify these as non-medical expenses.

[b] A CMS official we spoke with stated that revenues were higher than projected because MA organizations received additional payments to compensate for enrollees who were potentially more costly because of severity of illness, were disproportionately from counties with higher benchmarks, were disproportionately enrolled in more expensive plans, or a combination of the three.

Table 2. Actual and Projected Medical Expenses, Non-Medical Expenses, and Profits as Amounts and Percentages of Revenue among HMOs, PPOs, and PFFS, 2006

	Actual		Projected		Difference between actual and projected	
	Percentage of revenue	Amount in dollars (billions)	Percentage of revenue	Amount in dollars (billions)	Percentage of revenue	Amount in dollars (billions)
HMOs Contracts = 165 Beneficiaries = 4,606,255						
Medical expenses[a]	83.4	35.74	86.8	35.57	-3.4	0.18
Non-medical expenses	9.4	4.01	8.7	3.58	0.6	0.42
Profits	7.2	3.10	4.4	1.82	2.8	1.28
PPOs Contracts = 42 Beneficiaries = 238,258						
Medical expenses[a]	85.5	1.83	88.0	1.94	-2.5	-0.11
Non-medical expenses	10.5	0.23	9.4	0.21	1.2	0.02
Profits	4.0	0.08	2.7	0.06	1.3	0.03
PFFS Contracts = 10 Beneficiaries = 635,126						
Medical expenses[a]	81.3	3.86	87.7	4.23	-6.4	-0.37
Non-medical expenses	15.6	0.74	10.0	0.48	5.6	0.26
Profits	3.1	0.15	2.3	0.11	0.8	0.04

Source: CMS.

Notes: Data on actual expenses and profits were self-reported by MA organizations. Percentages are weighted by total revenue. Percentage totals may add to more or less than 100 due to rounding. We did not include regional PPOs in the PPO category. We excluded from our analysis employer group health plans and contracts for which revenue projections or actual expenditures were not reported. We also excluded from our analysis contracts that had fewer than 24,000 member months, which is equivalent to 2,000 beneficiaries enrolled for a full year. We reported enrollment by plan type in terms of the number of beneficiaries; each beneficiary is equivalent to 12 member months. The analysis includes 217 contracts, representing about 55 percent of the contracts for which a two-year look-back form was submitted and about 82 percent of

MA enrollment, equivalent to approximately 5.5 million beneficiaries enrolled in contracted plans for a full year.

[a]A CMS official we spoke with stated that medical expenses as a percentage of revenue may vary for reasons other than utilization and cost of providing care. Some MA organizations, for example, may categorize the costs of care management services as medical expenses, while other MA organizations may classify these as non-medical expenses.

Table 3. Actual Medical Expenses, Non-Medical Expenses, and Profits as Amounts and Percentages of Revenue, 2005 and 2006

	2005			2006		
	Percentage of revenue	**Amount in dollars per beneficiary**	**Amount in dollars (billions)**	**Percentage of revenue**	**Amount in dollars per beneficiary**	**Amount in dollars (billions)**
Medical expenses[a]	85.9	7,749.66	30.06	83.3	7,551.38	42.15
Non-medical expenses	9.2	827.72	3.21	10.1	913.59	5.10
Profits	5.0	448.12	1.74	6.6	601.79	3.36
Total Revenue		**9,025.50**	**35.01**		**9,066.76**	**50.61**

Source: CMS.

Notes: Data on actual expenses and profits were self-reported by MA organizations. Percentages for 2005 and 2006 are weighted by 2005 and 2006 total revenue, respectively. Percentage totals may add to more than 100 due to rounding. We excluded from our analysis employer group health plans and contracts for which revenue projections or actual expenditures were not reported. We also excluded from our analysis contracts that had fewer than 24,000 member months, which is equivalent to 2,000 beneficiaries enrolled for a full year. The 2005 analysis includes 120 contracts, representing about 81 percent of the contracts for which a two-year look-back form was submitted and about 78 percent of MA enrollment, equivalent to approximately 3.9 million beneficiaries enrolled in contracted plans for a full year. The 2006 analysis includes 224 contracts, representing about 57 percent of the contracts for which a two-year look-back form was submitted and about 84 percent of MA enrollment, equivalent to approximately 5.6 million beneficiaries enrolled in contracted plans for a full year.

[a]A CMS official we spoke with stated that medical expenses as a percentage of revenue may vary for reasons other than utilization and cost of providing care. Some MA organizations, for example, may categorize the costs of delivering care management services as medical expenses, while other MA organizations may classify these as non-medical expenses.

AGENCY COMMENTS

In commenting on a draft of our report, CMS stated that it agreed with our findings. In addition, CMS stated that the small difference between MA organizations' actual and projected aggregate medical expenses was within the prevailing range of such differences for a one-year-ahead estimate. CMS further noted that MA organizations' higher-than-projected profits were due primarily to higher-than-projected revenues from Medicare, and that the increase in revenues was at least partially due to higher-than-projected risk scores, reflecting enrollees who were deemed potentially more costly because of their health status.

We stated in our report that MA organizations self-reported spending only slightly less on medical expenses than projected; however, they received $1.7 billion more in revenues than projected. If MA organizations had more accurately projected both their revenues and expenses, they would have been able to provide beneficiaries with additional benefits or costsharing reductions, and still maintain the level of profits projected.

As agreed with your office, unless you publicly announce its contents earlier, we plan no further distribution of this report until 30 days from its date. At that time, we will send copies of this report to the Acting Administrator of CMS and relevant congressional committees and other interested members. The report will also be available at no charge on the GAO Web site at http://www.gao.gov.

If you or your staff have any questions regarding this report, please contact me at (202) 512-7114 or cosgrovej@gao.gov. Contact points for our Offices of Congressional Relations and Public Affairs may be found on the last page of this report. Christine Brudevold, Assistant Director; Gregory Giusto; Dan Lee; and Jessica T. Lee were major contributors to this report.

Sincerely yours,

James C. Cosgrove
Director, Health Care
Enclosure

ENCLOSURE I

Comments from the Centers for Medicare & Medicaid Services

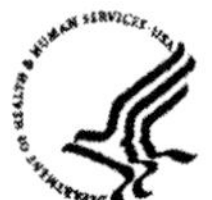

DEPARTMENT OF HEALTH & HUMAN SERVICES OFFICE OF THE SECRETARY

Assistant Secretary for Legislation
Washington, DC 20201

DEC 02 2008

James Cosgrove
Director, Health Care
U.S. Government Accountability Office
441 G Street, NW
Washington, DC 20548

Dear Mr. Cosgrove:

Enclosed are the Department's comments on the U.S. Government Accountability Office's (GAO) draft report entitled: "Medicare Advantage Organizations: Actual Expenses and Profits Compared to Projections" (GAO 09-132R).

The Department appreciates the opportunity to comment on this draft report before its publication.

Sincerely,

Jennifer R. Luong
for Vincent J. Ventimiglia, Jr.
Assistant Secretary for Legislation

Attachment

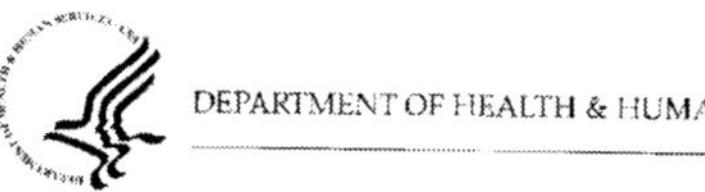

Centers for Medicare & Medicaid Services

200 Independence Avenue SW
Washington, DC 20201

DATE: DEC 0 2 2008

TO: Vincent J. Ventimiglia, Jr.
Assistant Secretary for Legislation
Department of Health and Human Services

FROM: Kerry Weems
Acting Administrator

SUBJECT: Government Accountability Office (GAO) Draft Correspondence: "Medicare Advantage Organizations: Actual Expenses and Profits Compared to Projections" (GAO-09-132R)

Thank you for the opportunity to review and comment on the GAO correspondence entitled, "Draft Correspondence: Medicare Advantage Organizations: Actual Expenses and Profits Compared to Projections." While CMS agrees with the findings set forth in this draft report, we have one comment.

As illustrated in Table 1, the aggregate actual medical expenses were within one percent of projected. The very small difference shown in this comparison is significant because of the inherent variability in medical trends and difficulty in forecasting medical spending—the result is well within the prevailing range of such differences for a one-year-ahead estimate. Further, it appears that the primary reason actual profit margins were higher than projected is that plans received greater revenue than projected. Projections of plan revenue, which are included in plan bids, were based in part on projected risk scores, which were lower than the subsequent actual risk scores. Since actual risk scores were greater than projected, plans received greater revenue than projected based on these risk scores.

Again, CMS appreciates the opportunity to review and comment on this draft report.

End Notes

[1] Statement of Peter R. Orszag, Congressional Budget Office, *The Medicare Advantage Program: Enrollment Trends and Budgetary Effects*, testimony before the Senate Committee on Finance, April 11, 2007.

[2] Medicare is the federally financed health insurance program for persons aged 65 and over, certain individuals with disabilities, and individuals with end-stage renal disease. Medicare Part A covers hospital and other inpatient stays. Medicare Part B is optional insurance, and covers hospital outpatient, physician, and other services. Medicare Parts A and B are known as original Medicare or Medicare FFS. Medicare beneficiaries have the option of obtaining coverage for Medicare Parts A and B services from private health plans that participate in Medicare's MA program—also known as Medicare Part C. All Medicare beneficiaries are eligible for coverage for outpatient prescription drugs under Medicare Part D.

[3] However, payments to MA organizations may be modified based on differences in actual and projected beneficiary health status, beneficiary residence, and enrollment. Actual expenses may be used to inform projections for future contract years.

[4] See GAO, *Medicare Advantage Organizations: Actual Expenses and Profits Compared to Projections for 2005*, GAO-08-827R (Washington, D.C.: June 24, 2008). Prior to 2006, private health plans provided health coverage to Medicare beneficiaries through the Medicare + Choice program. The Medicare Prescription Drug, Improvement, and Modernization Act of 2003 renamed that program "Medicare Advantage" among other changes. Pub. L. No. 108-173, § 201, 117 Stat. 2066, 2176. Organizations were required to begin using the new program name in 2006, but CMS encouraged MA organizations to transition to "Medicare Advantage" in all plan materials for the 2005 contract year.

[5] MA organizations are required to submit bids annually for review and approval for each plan they intend to offer. The bid submission includes a Bid Pricing Tool, which contains MA organizations' projections of their revenue requirements and revenue sources.

[6] The two-year look-back form is so named because it provides data for the calendar year 2 years prior to the upcoming contract year. The two-year look-back form was not certified by the MA plan's actuary in 2008.

[7] "Member months" is the sum of a given contract's total monthly enrollments in a year. For example, if 1,500 members were enrolled in an organization's plan for January and February and 2,000 members were enrolled in its plans for March through December, the contract would have 23,000 member months. Contracts with relatively low enrollments are not credible because their expenses can be unduly affected by outlier cases.

[8] While each contract may include more than one health benefit plan, each contract is designated as having only one plan type. Beneficiaries in HMOs are generally restricted to seeing providers within a network, while PFFS beneficiaries can see any provider that accepts the plan's payment terms. Beneficiaries in PPOs can see both in-network and out-of-network providers but must pay higher costsharing amounts if they use out-of-network services. We did not include regional PPOs in the PPO category.

[9] Before July 1, 2001, CMS was known as the Health Care Financing Administration.

[10] Profits or profit margins refer to MA organizations' remaining revenue after medical and non-medical expenses are paid. Profits may include other revenue offsets that are not captured in the non-medical expenses category, such as income taxes. In certain circumstances, such as for new market entrants, CMS allows MA organizations to have a negative profit, meaning that the organization's revenue is less than its combined medical and non-medical expenses.

[11] See GAO, *Medicare Advantage: Increased Spending Relative to Medicare Fee-for-Service May Not Always Reduce Beneficiary Out-of-Pocket Costs*, GAO-08-359 (Washington, D.C.: Feb. 22, 2008).

[12] GAO-08-827R.

[13] There were several large outlier contracts whose relatively large difference between actual and projected profits made up more than half of the $1.1 billion difference.

[14] To adjust for any misestimates of the number of enrolled beneficiaries, we multiplied both actual and projected per member per month revenues and profits by actual 2006 enrollment.

[15] CMS assigns Medicare enrollees a health status score based on their diagnoses and demographic characteristics. MA organizations are paid more for beneficiaries who are expected to need more care or more expensive care.

[16] Under the payment system in 2005, MA organizations were paid an administrative set rate regardless of their projections. If an MA organization's projection was less than the administratively set rate, the organization was required to spend the surplus Medicare payment on beneficiaries by adding extra benefits, reducing beneficiary cost sharing, or contributing to a benefit stabilization fund.

[17] In an ordered set of values, the median is a value below and above which there is an equal number of values; if there is no one middle number, it is the arithmetic mean (average) of the two middle values.

In: Medicare Advantage: The Alternate Medicare … ISBN: 978-1-60876-031-2
Editors: Charles V. Baylis, pp.149-159

Chapter 5

MEDICARE ADVANTAGE: PRIVATE HEALTH PLANS IN MEDICARE

Congressional Budget Office

Medicare provides federal health insurance for 43 million people who are aged or disabled or who have end-stage renal disease. Most receive services through the traditional fee-for-service (FFS) part of the program, which pays providers a set fee for each covered service (or bundle of services). Participants can choose their providers and are not required to obtain prior authorization for any covered service.

Medicare beneficiaries have the option of enrolling in Medicare Advantage—the program through which private plans participate in Medicare—rather than receiving their care through the FFS program.[1] They may choose to do so because such plans provide additional benefits beyond those available within traditional Medicare, including coverage for services not covered by FFS Medicare (for instance, dental services) and cash rebates of premiums or reduced cost-sharing. As of June 2007, about 18 percent of beneficiaries are enrolled in Medicare Advantage plans.[2] This brief describes how those private plans function, how they are paid, how their costs compare with the costs of traditional Medicare, and how those costs vary by geographic area.

In summary:

- Enrollment in Medicare Advantage is growing rapidly, particularly in a relatively unmanaged type of plan called private fee for service (PFFS).

- Medicare's payments for beneficiaries enrolled in Medicare Advantage plans are higher, on average, than what the program would spend if those beneficiaries were in the FFS sector—so shifts in enrollment out of the FFS program and into private plans increase net Medicare spending.
- The difference in costs relative to those for the traditional FFS program is particularly large for PFFS plans.
- The additional cost to the government for Medicare Advantage plans subsidizes the beneficiaries who enroll in such plans, which fuels the plans' growth in enrollment and raises costs for Medicare beneficiaries who do not participate in Medicare Advantage.
- Reducing the payment differential between Medicare Advantage and the FFS program could result in substantial savings to the Medicare program. But it would also diminish the supplemental benefits and cash rebates that Medicare Advantage plans can offer to enrollees and lessen enrollment in those plans. Lowering payments to those plans would slightly reduce the standard premiums for Part B of Medicare (Supplementary Medical Insurance) and delay the exhaustion of the trust fund that supports Part A (Hospital Insurance).

Types of Medicare Advantage Plans

About 80 percent of beneficiaries currently enrolled in the Medicare Advantage program are in health maintenance organizations (HMOs) or preferred provider organizations (PPOs). Both HMOs and PPOs have comprehensive networks of providers, but PPOs allow beneficiaries to obtain care outside the network if they pay higher amounts.[3] A key feature of many HMO and PPO plans is care management services, which are intended to promote better coordination and moreeffective use of health care, although little evidence exists on whether HMO and PPO plans succeed in delivering higher-quality care than traditional Medicare.

The other main type of Medicare Advantage plan is private fee for service. Such plans allow their enrollees to obtain care from any provider who will furnish it and are not required to maintain networks of providers. In contrast to the FFS system, which requires participating providers to accept Medicare's rates for all covered services and all beneficiaries, providers in a PFFS plan can decide each time they see a patient whether to accept the plan's terms of participation and payment rates, which are usually those of Medicare's FFS program. Beneficiaries' premiums, copayments, and deductibles are generally lower than those in the FFS program, and private fee-for-service plans typically provide significantly less care management and utilization control than do HMOs and PPOs (see Box 1).

BOX 1. HOW MEDICARE ADVANTAGE PLANS ARE PAID

The current payment system for private health plans was established by the Medicare Modernization Act, which was enacted in 2003.[1] Private plans that want to participate in the Medicare Advantage program must submit bids indicating the per capita payment for which they are willing to provide Medicare's Part A (Hospital Insurance) and Part B (Supplementary Medical Insurance) benefits—and to take on the financial risk of doing so.[2]

The government compares those bids with county-level benchmarks that are determined in advance through statutory rules. The benchmarks are the maximum payment the government will make for enrollees in private plans; in most cases the plans' bids (and the resulting payments) are lower than the benchmarks. (The benchmark for a plan that serves more than one county is an enrollment-weighted average of the county-level benchmarks in its service area.)

If a plan's bid is less than the benchmark, Medicare pays the plan its bid plus 75 percent of the amount by which the benchmark exceeds the bid. Such a plan must return that 75 percent to beneficiaries as additional benefits or as a rebate of their Part B or Part D premiums.[3] For example, if a county's benchmark is $800 per person per month and a plan bids $700, Medicare will pay the plan $775, and $75 of that amount must be returned in some form to the beneficiaries. Such additional benefits and lower premiums are a primary factor distinguishing one Medicare Advantage plan from another and Medicare Advantage plans from Medicare's fee-for-service (FFS) program.

Benchmarks are required to be at least as high as per capita expenditures in the FFS program in every county and are higher than FFS expenditures in many counties. For 2007, the Congressional Budget Office calculates that benchmarks are 17 percent higher, on average, than projected per capita FFS expenditures nationwide. Benchmarks are updated each year by either the growth in national per capita Medicare spending or 2 percent, whichever is greater. For 2008, the benchmarks will increase by 3.5 percent.

Medicare also adjusts payments to Medicare Advantage plans to reflect their enrollees' health status. That "risk adjustment" is meant to encourage plans to compete on the basis of efficient delivery of services rather than selective enrollment of healthier beneficiaries. To that end, the Centers for Medicare & Medicaid Services (CMS) collects information on the medical diagnoses of every beneficiary in the FFS and Medicare Advantage programs and uses it to calculate the relationship between individuals' health and subsequent spending on their behalf for Medicare services and to thereby adjust payments to plans (upward for those with sicker beneficiaries and downward for those with healthier beneficiaries).

In managing the risk adjustment system, CMS has to confront difficult issues of data collection and validity, statistical complexity, and potentially different coding practices among plans and the FFS sector. Each judgment the agency makes for each of those aspects of risk adjustment can increase or decrease payments to Medicare Advantage plans.

1. The description of the payment mechanism in this box pertains to plans that participate in Medicare on a county-bycounty basis (or "local" plans). The mechanism for regional preferred provider organizations is analogous to that described here for local plans but uses a modified approach to compute benchmarks. See Medicare Payment Advisory Commission, Report to the Congress: Issues in a Modernized Medicare Program (June 2005), pp. 59–81.
2. Part A covers inpatient services provided by hospitals as well as skilled nursing and hospice care. Part B covers services provided by physicians and other practitioners, hospitals' outpatient departments, and suppliers of medical equipment.
3. If a plan's bid is above the benchmark, Medicare pays the bid amount, and the plan is required to charge enrollees the difference between the bid and what Medicare pays.

In 2007, 82 percent of Medicare beneficiaries live in a county served by an HMO or a local PPO, up from 67 percent in 2005.[4] All beneficiaries have access to a PFFS plan in 2007, up from 80 percent in 2006 and only 45 percent in 2005. Most Medicare beneficiaries have access to more than one private plan.

Enrollment in Medicare Advantage Plans Is Increasing Rapidly

Enrollment in Medicare Advantage plans has grown rapidly in recent years. In 2003 and 2004, Medicare Advantage plans accounted for 11 percent of enrollment in Medicare, the lowest level since 1996. Over the past two years, however, enrollment in those health plans has increased to about 18 percent of all enrollment, or 8 million beneficiaries. That increase reflects, among other factors, changes enacted in the Medicare Modernization Act that increased payment rates and added the prescription drug benefit to complement the medical benefits provided under Parts A and B of Medicare.[5] The Congressional Budget Office (CBO) projects that, under current law, enrollment in Medicare Advantage will grow at an annual average rate of about 7 percent over the next 10 years, compared with a growth rate of about 2.5 percent for Medicare overall—reaching 21 percent of total enrollment in 2008 and 26 percent by 2017 (see Figure 1).

The projected increase in enrollment in Medicare Advantage is driven largely by CBO's expectation of continuing growth in enrollment in private fee-for-service plans, which rose from 200,000 members at the end of 2005 to more than 1.6 million members in June 2007—about 700,000 of whom were added during 2007. By 2017, CBO anticipates, enrollment in PFFS plans will reach 5 million members, accounting for one-third of all Medicare Advantage enrollment at that time, up from about one-fifth now.

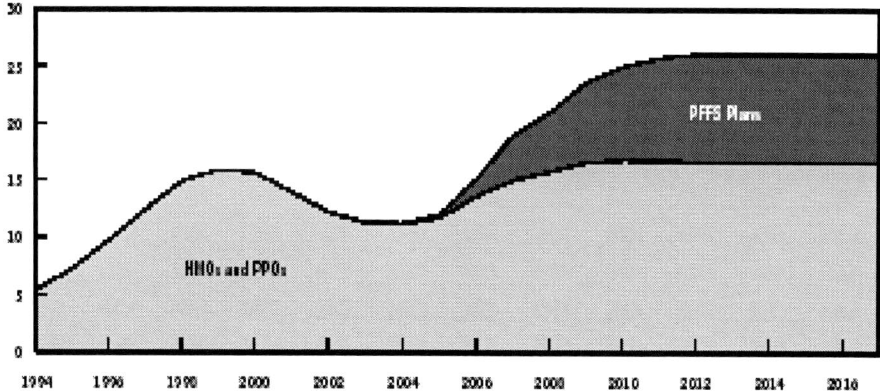

Source: Congressional Budget Office.

Notes: HMO = health maintenance organization; PPO = preferred provider organization; PFFS = private fee for service. For the purpose of this figure, enrollment in Medicare is considered to be that in Part A (Hospital Insurance).

Figure 1. Enrollment in Medicare Advantage as a Percentage of Enrollment in Medicare

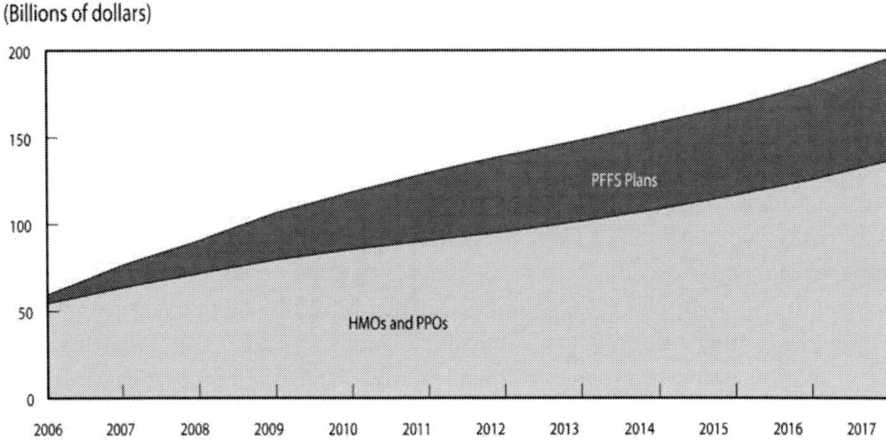

Source: Congressional Budget Office.

Note: HMO = health maintenance organization; PPO = preferred provider organization; PFFS = private fee for service.

Figure 2. Projected Spending on Medicare Advantage, by Type of Plan

SPENDING ON MEDICARE ADVANTAGE IS RISING

CBO projects that, under current law, payments to Medicare Advantage plans for benefits under Parts A and B will rise from $60 billion in 2006 to $196 billion in 2017—reflecting an annual average growth rate of 11 percent (see Figure 2).[6] Much of that increase (about 7 percent per year) will result from growing enrollment; the rest (about 4 percent per year), from increasing payments per enrollee. By comparison, CBO estimates that total enrollment in Medicare will grow much more slowly and that total spending will increase by an average of 6.5 percent per year. Spending for Medicare Advantage is projected to total approximately $1.5 trillion from 2007 through 2017, more than a quarter of all spending for benefits under Parts A and B.

CBO expects that private fee-for-service plans will account for a rapidly growing share of Medicare Advantage spending under current law, with payments to them increasing from approximately $5 billion in 2006 to $13 billion in 2007 and $59 billion in 2017. That increase represents an annual average nominal growth rate of 25 percent over the 11-year period, reflecting a 20 percent average rate of growth in enrollment. In 2006, PFFS plans accounted for approximately 8 percent of Medicare Advantage spending; in 2017, CBO anticipates, those plans will account for about 30 percent. Although they are expected to grow more slowly than PFFS plans, HMOs and PPOs are likely to continue to account for the largest portion of spending throughout the coming decade.

MEDICARE ADVANTAGE PLANS COST THE GOVERNMENT MORE THAN TRADITIONAL MEDICARE

The government's spending for beneficiaries in Medicare Advantage plans will, in almost all cases, exceed what it would spend if those beneficiaries were in the traditional fee-for-service sector. That outcome occurs because benchmarks are almost always higher than FFS costs, and the government retains only 25 percent of the difference between a plan's bid and the benchmark.

In 2007, CBO estimates, the average payment to such plans is 12 percent above traditional FFS costs.7 The differential is larger for private fee-for-service plans: According to estimates by the Medicare Payment Advisory Commission (MedPAC), the payments to those plans in 2006 averaged 19 percent above FFS costs.[8] Of that difference, 10 percentage points' worth went to beneficiaries in the form of extra benefits or rebates. In contrast, payments to HMOs averaged 10 percent above FFS costs, MedPAC estimates. On average, HMOs offered extra benefits and rebates equal to 13 percent of FFS costs; those additional benefits and rebates reflected the difference between the benchmark (which averaged 10 percent above FFS costs) and the plans' bids (which averaged 3 percent below FFS costs).

The extra benefits and rebates offered by Medicare Advantage plans attract enrollees, and the rising proportion of beneficiaries enrolling in the plans will add to the growth in Medicare spending. In addition, because premiums for Part B of Medicare are set to cover 25 percent of the costs of that program, the higher costs of Medicare Advantage plans add about $2 to the monthly premium for Part B.[9] Those higher costs also accelerate the exhaustion of the trust fund that supports Part A.

Private plans can provide the services of Parts A and B at a lower cost than the FFS program can only if they offset their higher administrative costs by achieving savings through lower utilization of services or smaller payments to providers. In general, HMOs keep their medical costs down by reducing the level and intensity of utilization, particularly by limiting their enrollees' use of services such as visits to specialists, inpatient hospital care, costly tests and procedures, and services in intensive care units.[10] In contrast to HMOs and PPOs, private fee-for-service plans generally do not incur the costs of establishing and maintaining networks of providers, and the rates paid to providers by PFFS plans generally are the same as Medicare's FFS costs. PFFS plans also incur administrative costs for acquiring and maintaining enrollment, but they do not realize comparable savings from managing utilization. In a given area, differences between the costs incurred by various Medicare Advantage plans may not substantially affect the government's costs, however, because in most cases, three-quarters of any savings accrues to beneficiaries.

ENROLLMENT IN MEDICARE ADVANTAGE VARIES GEOGRAPHICALLY

Most enrollment in HMOs and PPOs tends to be in relatively densely populated areas (where establishing provider networks is easier) with relatively high benchmarks and generally high per capita FFS spending.[11] Because those types of private plans try to restrain medical costs by managing the utilization of services, they have a greater potential to achieve savings relative to the FFS program in areas where FFS practice involves relatively high utilization of costly services. (To the extent that such cost savings are realized, they should be reflected in future bids and thus lead to expanded benefits for Medicare Advantage enrollees, with a quarter of the savings returned to the Medicare program.) HMOs and PPOs have much less opportunity to achieve such savings in areas where the utilization of expensive services in the FFS sector is already relatively low.

In contrast to HMOs and PPOs, private fee-for service plans have enrollment that is far more dispersed, including significant enrollment in rural areas. The rapid growth of those plans increased the market share of private plans in rural areas from about 4 percent in 2005 to about 7 percent in 2006, and CBO expects that share to continue to grow under current law as PFFS plans play an increasingly large role in Medicare Advantage. They are able to grow in rural areas, first, because they face little competition from other types of private plans there; unlike HMOs and PPOs, they do not require networks of providers, which are difficult to establish in those areas. Second, Medicare rules enable private fee-for-service plans to pay providers at the same rates as FFS Medicare does, which are generally lower than the rates that HMOs and PPOs negotiate with providers that join their networks. Finally, benchmarks in rural areas are sufficiently high that PFFS plans are able to offer extra benefits or rebates to attract members even without the cost-reducing tools available to other types of plans.

THE IMPACT OF REDUCING PAYMENTS TO MEDICARE ADVANTAGE PLANS

All counties have benchmarks set at or above local per capita FFS spending. On average, benchmarks are 17 percent higher, CBO calculates. By CBO's estimates, more than one-half of Medicare Advantage spending is in counties where the benchmark is at least 10 percent above FFS costs, and more than one-fifth is in counties where the benchmark is 20 percent higher or more (see Table 1). Reducing benchmarks to FFS levels would therefore constitute a significant reduction in spending in most counties. Relative to spending under current law, CBO estimates, that policy would save $54 billion over the 2009–2012 period and $149 billion over the 2009–2017 period.[12] Limiting benchmarks to 100 percent of FFS costs for private fee-for-service plans and maintaining current-law benchmarks for other plans would reduce federal spending by about $14 billion over the 2009– 2012 period and $43 billion over the 2009–2017 period. Each policy would, however, have a considerable impact on both plans and their participants.

Much of the benefit of the higher benchmarks accrues to participants in the plans in the form of supplemental benefits or lower premiums, and reducing benchmarks would leave less money for those purposes. (In the example cited in the box, with a benchmark of $800 and a plan's bid of $700, if per capita FFS spending in the county averaged $660, setting payments to the plan at the FFS average would reduce the government's costs from $775 to $660 per person; at least $75 of that reduction would be reflected as reduced benefits or increased costs to the plan's participants.) Such a change, in turn, would make the program less attractive to beneficiaries and lead some to return to the traditional fee-for-service program. Others who would have joined Medicare Advantage plans would remain in the FFS program.

The change also would make the Medicare Advantage program less attractive for health plans and cause some to leave the program, as they did after the Congress constrained increases in payment rates in the Balanced Budget Act of 1997. By CBO's estimates, setting benchmarks to FFS levels would reduce enrollment in Medicare Advantage by about 6.2 million beneficiaries in 2012 relative to the agency's baseline projection, a decline of about 50 percent from the projected level of 12.5 million in 2012 and about 1.7 million relative to today's enrollment. Limiting the policy change to private fee-for-service plans would result in a smaller reduction in enrollment, approximately 3.3 million beneficiaries in 2012.

Some types of plans and some areas would be affected more than others. Under both options, PFFS plans, which generally receive the highest per capita payments relative to FFS costs, would be affected more than HMOs and PPOs. Rural areas would be affected more than urban ones. And some states would be affected more than others; on average, the benchmarks exceed FFS costs by as little as 6 percent in Connecticut but by as much as 41 percent in Hawaii.[13] Lowering the benchmarks would also delay the exhaustion of the Hospital Insurance trust fund, and slightly reduce the standard Part B premiums.

Table 1. Distribution of Medicare Advantage Spending, by the Percentage by Which County Benchmarks Exceed Local FFS per Capita Costs

Percent		
Percentage by Which Benchmark Exceeds FFS Costs	**Portion of Medicare Advantage Spending**	
	Within Category	**Within or Above Category**
0	10	100
Greater Than 0 to 9.9	38	90
10 to 19.9	31	52
20 to 29.9	12	21
30 to 39.9	5	9
40 to 49.9	1	4
50 and Higher	3	3

Source: Congressional Budget Office.

Note: Categories are based on the Medicare Advantage program's local county benchmarks and local fee-for-service (FFS) rates. The total spending is calculated as if all bids were equal to the benchmark and all beneficiaries had average expected costs. The analysis includes all counties with reported FFS spending for 2007 (as well as Puerto Rico).

End Notes

[1]Medicare Advantage is also called Part C. Previously, the program had been called Medicare+Choice.

[2] Another 1 percent of beneficiaries are enrolled in other types of group plans, including cost-reimbursed plans, health care prepayment plans, a program of all-inclusive care for the elderly, and demonstration plans.

[3] PPOs in the Medicare Advantage program are either local or regional; regional PPOs, an option that became available in 2006, are required to serve broad regions of the country rather than defining their service areas on a county-by-county basis. About 2 percent of Medicare Advantage beneficiaries are enrolled in regional PPOs.

[4] See Medicare Payment Advisory Commission, *Report to the Congress: Medicare Payment Policy* (March 2007), Chapter 4, "Update on Medicare Private Plans," pp. 237–266.

[5] Part A, Hospital Insurance, covers inpatient services provided by hospitals as well as skilled nursing and hospice care. Part B, Supplementary Medical Insurance, covers services provided by physicians and other practitioners, hospitals' outpatient departments, and suppliers of medical equipment. Home health care may be covered by either Part A or Part B. Health maintenance organizations and preferred provider organizations must offer a prescription drug benefit under Part D; they may choose to also offer an option that does not include that benefit. Plans must submit separate bids for the prescription drug benefit and identify the premiums they intend to charge for any supplemental benefits they offer.

[6] Excluded here are payments for Part D benefits, which are managed separately.

[7] In areas with high FFS costs per capita, benchmarks and plans' bids tend to be closer to FFS spending; in areas with low FFS costs, benchmarks and bids diverge more from FFS spending. In particular, in areas with the highest FFS spending, health plans' bids for 2007 are about 9 percent *below* FFS spending; benchmark rates in those areas average about 4 percent *above* FFS costs. By contrast, in the lowest-cost FFS areas, health plans' bids are about 16 percent *above* FFS spending, and benchmark rates average about 26 percent *above* FFS costs. For further discussion, see Congressional Budget Office, *Designing a Premium Support System for Medicare* (December 2006).

[8] Statement of Glen M. Hackbarth, Chairman, Medicare Payment Advisory Commission, *The Medicare Advantage Program and MedPAC Recommendations,* before the Senate Committee on Finance (April 11, 2007), p. 5.

[9] Ibid.

[10] See Robert H. Miller and Harold S. Luft, "HMO Plan Performance Update: An Analysis of the Literature, 1997-2001," *Health Affairs*, vol. 21, no. 4 (July/August 2002), pp. 63–86.

[11] It is easier for a plan to establish a network in a relatively densely populated area that has a relatively large number of providers than in a more sparsely populated area because the plan's leverage in negotiations with providers (to get them to accept lower payment rates and to cooperate with the plan's efforts to manage utilization) relies on promising them some volume of business by diverting to them patients from providers who do not participate in the network.

[12] The county-level benchmarks for 2008 have been announced, and the bidding process is under way. CBO's estimates assume that the policy would take effect in 2009 to avoid interrupting the bidding process for 2008. There are numerous other policy options for reducing payments to Medicare Advantage plans; for some of those and their estimated budgetary impact, see Statement of Peter R. Orszag, Director, Congressional Budget Office, *The Medicare Advantage Program,* before the House Committee on the Budget (June 28, 2007), Tables 4 and 5, pp. 16–20.

[13] See Congressional Budget Office, *Medicare Advantage Statistics by State* (April 17, 2007).

CHAPTER SOURCES

The following chapters have been previously published:

Chapter 1 – This is an edited, excerpted and augmented edition of a United States Congressional Research Service publication, Report Order Code R40374, dated March 3, 2009.

Chapter 2 – This This is an edited, excerpted and augmented edition of a United States Government Accountability Office (GAO), Report to Congressional Requestors. Publication GAO-09-25, dated December 2008.

Chapter 3 – This This is an edited, excerpted and augmented edition of a United States Government Accountability Office (GAO), Report to Congressional Requestors. Publication GAO-08-359, dated February 2008.

Chapter 4 - This This is an edited, excerpted and augmented edition of a United States Government Accountability Office (GAO), Report to Congressional Requestors. Publication GAO-09-132R, dated December 2008.

Chapter 5 – This is an edited, excerpted and augmented edition of a United States Congressional Budget Office, Economic and Budget Issue Brief, dated June 28, 2007.

INDEX

E

F

G

H

P

Q

R

S

T

U

V

X